C000051528

Controversies in Hepatology

The Experts Analyze Both Sides

Controversies in Hepatology

The Experts Analyze Both Sides

Donald M. Jensen, MD
Professor of Medicine
Director, Center for Liver Diseases
University of Chicago Medical Center
Chicago, Illinois

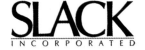

www.slackbooks.com

ISBN: 978-1-55642-950-7

Copyright © 2011 by SLACK Incorporated

All rights reserved. No part of this book may be reproduced, stored in a retrieval system or transmitted in any form or by any means, electronic, mechanical, photocopying, recording or otherwise, without written permission from the publisher, except for brief quotations embodied in critical articles and reviews.

The procedures and practices described in this book should be implemented in a manner consistent with the professional standards set for the circumstances that apply in each specific situation. Every effort has been made to confirm the accuracy of the information presented and to correctly relate generally accepted practices. The authors, editor, and publisher cannot accept responsibility for errors or exclusions or for the outcome of the material presented herein. There is no expressed or implied warranty of this book or information imparted by it. Care has been taken to ensure that drug selection and dosages are in accordance with currently accepted/recommended practice. Off-label uses of drugs may be discussed. Due to continuing research, changes in government policy and regulations, and various effects of drug reactions and interactions, it is recommended that the reader carefully review all materials and literature provided for each drug, especially those that are new or not frequently used. Any review or mention of specific companies or products is not intended as an endorsement by the author or publisher.

SLACK Incorporated uses a review process to evaluate submitted material. Prior to publication, educators or clinicians provide important feedback on the content that we publish. We welcome feedback on this work.

Published by: SLACK Incorporated
                6900 Grove Road
                Thorofare, NJ 08086 USA
                Telephone: 856-848-1000
                Fax: 856-848-6091
                www.slackbooks.com

Contact SLACK Incorporated for more information about other books in this field or about the availability of our books from distributors outside the United States.

Library of Congress Cataloging-in-Publication Data

Controversies in hepatology : the experts analyze both sides / [edited by] Donald M. Jensen.
    p. ; cm.
  Includes bibliographical references and index.
ISBN 978-1-55642-950-7 (pbk. : alk. paper) 1. Liver--Diseases--Treatment. 2. Decision making.
3. Evidence-based medicine. I. Jensen, Donald.
  [DNLM: 1. Liver Diseases--therapy. 2. Decision Making. 3. Evidence-Based Medicine. 4. Liver Diseases--diagnosis. WI 700]
  RC845.C64 2011
  616.3'6206--dc22
                                2011017339

For permission to reprint material in another publication, contact SLACK Incorporated. Authorization to photocopy items for internal, personal, or academic use is granted by SLACK Incorporated provided that the appropriate fee is paid directly to Copyright Clearance Center. Prior to photocopying items, please contact the Copyright Clearance Center at 222 Rosewood Drive, Danvers, MA 01923 USA; phone: 978-750-8400; web site: www.copyright.com; email: info@copyright.com

Printed in the United States of America.

Last digit is print number: 10   9   8   7   6   5   4   3   2   1

Dedication

This book is dedicated to my loving wife, Donna, and to our two terrific children, Colin and Emily. They keep my head from getting too big.

Contents

Dedication .... *v*
Acknowledgments .... *ix*
About the Editor .... *xi*
Contributing Authors .... *xiii*
Preface .... *xvii*
Foreword by Willis C. Maddrey, MD .... *xix*

SECTION I   ACUTE LIVER DISEASE 1

Chapter 1   Alcoholic Hepatitis: Pentoxifylline Versus Steroids 3
             Leila Gobejishvili, PhD; Neil Crittenden, MD; and Craig J. McClain, MD

Chapter 2   Is N-Acetylcysteine Effective in All Cases of Non-Acetaminophen
             Acute Liver Failure? 11
             A. James Hanje, MD; Anthony Michaels, MD; and William M. Lee, MD

Chapter 3   Should Living Donor Transplantation Be Considered
             in Adult Acute Liver Failure? 19
             *AnnMarie Liapakis, MD; Julia Wattacheril, MD, MPH; and
             Robert S. Brown Jr, MD, MPH*

SECTION II   CHRONIC HEPATITIS B AND C 31

Chapter 4   Do All Patients With Chronic Hepatitis B Who Are Treatment
             Candidates Need an Assessment of Fibrosis? 33
             Hector Nazario, MD; Carmen Landaverde, MD; and Robert Perrillo, MD

Chapter 5   Should the Decompensated Hepatitis C Cirrhotic Be
             Treated With Antiviral Therapy? 43
             Payam Afshar, MD; Jeffrey Weissman, MD; and Paul J. Pockros, MD

Chapter 6   Should Hepatitis C Be Treated in Patients With Chronic Kidney
             Disease Prior to Kidney Transplant? 51
             Andres F. Carrion, MD; Seth N. Sclair, MD; and Paul Martin, MD

Chapter 7   Retransplantation for Severe Recurrent Hepatitis C Virus and
             Previously Failed Pegylated-Interferon/Ribavirin Therapy 61
             Vandana Khungar, MD, MSc; Tyralee Goo, MD; and Fred Poordad, MD

Chapter 8   Does a Sustained Virologic Response at Week 72 Indicate
             a Cure in Chronic Hepatitis C Virus? 73
             *Andrew Aronsohn, MD; Arjmand R. Mufti, MD, MRCP; and
             Nancy Reau, MD*

SECTION III   LIVER TUMORS 81

Chapter 9   Should Living Donor Liver Transplantation Be an Option
             for Patients With Hepatocellular Carcinoma Beyond
             the Milan Criteria? 83
             *Brett E. Fortune, MD; Alvaro Martinez-Camacho, MD; and
             James R. Burton Jr, MD*

Chapter 10   Resect or Observe Asymptomatic Hepatic Adenoma? 93
Joseph Ahn, MD, MS; Anjana Pillai, MD; and Stanley Martin Cohen, MD

SECTION IV   OTHER CHRONIC LIVER DISEASES AND CIRRHOSIS...................101

Chapter 11   Strictly Adhere to the "6-Month Rule" for Recent History of Alcohol Abuse
in Potential Liver Transplant Candidates? 103
Parul Dureja Agarwal, MD and Michael Ronan Lucey, MD

Chapter 12   Should Liver Biopsy Be Performed in All Patients With Nonalcoholic
Fatty Liver Disease? 111
Neehar D. Parikh, MD; Lisa VanWagner, MD; and Mary E. Rinella, MD

Chapter 13   Should the Hepatic Venous Pressure Gradient Be
Sequentially Measured to Monitor Beta-Blocker Therapy
in the Prophylaxis of Variceal Hemorrhage? 123
Cristina Ripoll, MD; Puneeta Tandon, MD; and Guadalupe Garcia-Tsao, MD

Chapter 14   Standard Dose or Avoid Ursodiol Therapy in Primary Sclerosing
Cholangitis? 133
*Dr. JS Halliday, MBBS (Hons.), FRACP; Ashley Barnabas, MD; and
Roger W. Chapman, MD, FRCP*

Chapter 15   Annual Screening of Primary Sclerosing Cholangitis Patients for
Cholangiocarcinoma With Magnetic Resonance
Cholangiopancreatography and CA 19-9? 145
*Boris Blechacz, MD, PhD; Nataliya Razumilava, MD; and
Gregory J. Gores, MD*

Chapter 16   Lactulose or Rifaximin as First-Line Therapy for
Hepatic Encephalopathy? 153
*Tarek I. Abu-Rajab Tamimi, MD; Thomas A. Brown, MD; and
Kevin D. Mullen, MD*

Chapter 17   Autoimmune Hepatitis: Maintenance Therapy for All
Patients or Stop Treatment After Histologic Remission? 159
*Ami Shah Behara, MD, MS; Cynthia K. Lau, MD; and
David Hoffman Van Thiel, MD*

Financial Disclosures 167
Index 171

Acknowledgments

This book would not have been possible without the stimulating discussions in hallways and conference rooms with hundreds, if not thousands, of fellows, residents, and medical students over the past thirty years. Teaching medicine is incredibly rewarding but also quite challenging as we educators are looked up to as the font of all wisdom. Our "expert" status, however, is only as good as our last correct diagnosis. This book is a dedicated to these trainees who keep us honest.

I would also like to thank my friends and colleagues at the Center for Liver Diseases at the University of Chicago for their help in identifying controversial areas and honing the direction of this book. In particular, Dr. Nancy Reau, Dr. Helen Te, Dr. Gautham Reddy, Dr. Andrew Aronsohn, Dr. Arjimand Mufti, and Dr. Smruti Mohanty deserve a special acknowledgement.

Finally, Carrie Kotlar and her colleagues at SLACK have been tremendous in facilitating the timely publication of this book. It was Carrie who came up with the final concept and title, and for this I am extremely grateful.

About the Editor

Donald M. Jensen, MD is Professor of Medicine, and Director of the Center for Liver Diseases, at the University of Chicago Medical Center. Dr. Jensen received his undergraduate (BS) and medical (MD) degrees from the University of Illinois in Urbana and Chicago, respectively. He completed a medicine internship and residency at Rush-Presbyterian-St. Luke's Medical Center in Chicago where he also served as Chief Medical Resident. After completing one year of gastroenterology fellowship at Rush, Dr. Jensen went to King's College Hospital in London, U.K., for a liver research fellowship under the mentorship of Professor Roger Williams. Returning to Chicago, Dr Jensen became a member of the Section of Digestive Diseases at Rush, specializing in clinical hepatology. In 1992, he became the Director, of the Section of Hepatology at Rush, and in 1999 the *Richard B. Capps* Professor of Medicine. In 2005, Dr. Jensen accepted his current position at the University of Chicago. He is board certified in both internal medicine and gastroenterology.

Dr. Jensen's research interest is in newer treatment strategies and therapies for hepatitis C. His clinical interests are broad and include: viral hepatitis, cirrhosis, autoimmune hepatitis and hepatocellular carcinoma, among others. He has authored or co-authored 74 peer-reviewed articles, 18 invited reviews/editorials, 23 book chapters, and 2 books (in preparation). He is a member of three editorial boards. He has been a member of the national board of directors of the American Liver Foundation (ALF); president of the Illinois chapter of the ALF; and is currently Treasurer and Governing Board member of the American Association for the Study of Liver Diseases (AASLD).

Dr. Jensen has received numerous teaching awards, including *Teacher of Year* on three occasions at both Rush University and the University of Chicago, as well as *Physician of the Year* award on two occasions from the ALF. He has been named *Top Doctor* by Chicago Magazine for the past 12 years, and is listed in *Who's Who in the World*. Dr. Jensen's hobbies include competitive running, swimming, and cycling and he has competed in 6 marathons, 12 triathlons and one Half Ironman triathlon. He is married to Dr. Donna Hanlon and they have two children, Colin and Emily.

Contributing Authors

Tarek I. Abu-Rajab Tamimi, MD (Chapter 16)
Department of Gastroenterology
Metrohealth Medical Center
Cleveland, Ohio

Payam Afshar, MD (Chapter 5)
Division of Gastroenterology/Hepatology
Scripps Clinic
San Diego, California

Parul Dureja Agarwal, MD (Chapter 11)
Transplant Hepatology Fellow
Division of Gastroenterology and
Hepatology
University of Wisconsin School of
Medicine and Public Health
Madison, Wisconsin

Joseph Ahn, MD, MS (Chapter 10)
Assistant Professor of Medicine
Medical Director, Liver Transplant
Loyola University Medical Center
Maywood, Illinois

Andrew Aronsohn, MD (Chapter 8)
Assistant Professor of Medicine
University of Chicago Medical Center
Center for Liver Diseases
Chicago, Illinois

Ashley Barnabas, MD (Chapter 14)
Specialist Registrar
John Radcliffe Hospital
Headington, Oxford, United Kingdom

Ami Shah Behara, MD, MS (Chapter 17)
Gastroenterology and Hepatology Fellow
Division of Gastroenterology and
Hepatology
Rush University Medical Center
Chicago, Illinois

Boris Blechacz, MD, PhD (Chapter 15)
Instructor in Medicine
Division of Gastroenterology and
Hepatology
Mayo Clinic
Rochester, Minnesota

Robert S. Brown Jr, MD, MPH (Chapter 3)
Frank Cardile Professor of Medicine
Chief, Center for Liver Disease &
Transplantation
Columbia University College of Physicians
& Surgeons
New York, New York

Thomas A. Brown, MD (Chapter 16)
Department of Gastroenterology
Metrohealth Medical Center
Cleveland, Ohio

James R. Burton Jr, MD (Chapter 9)
Medical Director of Liver Transplantation
Division of Gastroenterology and
Hepatology
University of Colorado Denver
Aurora, Colorado

Andres F. Carrion, MD (Chapter 6)
Department of Medicine
University of Miami
Miami, Florida

Roger W. Chapman, MD, FRCP (Chapter 14)
John Radcliffe Hospital
Translational Gastroenterology Unit,
Headington, Oxford, United Kingdom

Stanley Martin Cohen, MD (Chapter 10)
Director, Section of Hepatology
Associate Professor of Medicine
Loyola University Medical Center
Maywood, Illinois

Neil Crittenden, MD (Chapter 1)
Department of Medicine
University of Louisville School of
Medicine
Louisville, Kentucky

Brett E. Fortune, MD (Chapter 9)
Fellow, Division of Gastroenterology and
Hepatology
University of Colorado Denver
Aurora, Colorado

Guadalupe Garcia-Tsao, MD (Chapter 13)
Yale University School of Medicine
Digestive Diseases Section
New Haven, Connecticut

Leila Gobejishvili, PhD (Chapter 1)
Assistant Professor
Division of Gastroenterology, Hepatology,
and Nutrition
Alcohol Research Center; Department of
Medicine
University of Louisville School of Medicine
Louisville, Kentucky

Tyralee Goo, MD (Chapter 7)
Cedars-Sinai Medical Center
Department of Medicine
Los Angeles, California

Gregory J. Gores, MD (Chapter 15)
Reuben R. Eisenberg Professor of Medicine
Chair, Division of Gastroenterology and
Hepatology
Mayo Clinic
Rochester, Minnesota

JS Halliday, MBBS (Hons.), FRACP (Chapter 14)
John Radcliffe Hospital
Translational Gastroenterology Unit
Headington, Oxford, United Kingdom

A. James Hanje, MD (Chapter 2)
Assistant Professor of Medicine
The Ohio State University Medical Center
Columbus, Ohio

Vandana Khungar, MD, MSc (Chapter 7)
Fellow, David Geffen School of Medicine at
UCLA
Division of Gastroenterology
Los Angeles, California

Carmen Landaverde, MD (Chapter 4)
Baylor University Medical Center
Division of Hepatology
Dallas, Texas

Cynthia K. Lau, MD (Chapter 17)
Gastroenterology and Hepatology Fellow
Division of Gastroenterology and
Hepatology
Rush University Medical Center
Chicago, Illinois

William M. Lee, MD (Chapter 2)
Professor of Internal Medicine
University of Texas Southwestern Medical
Center at Dallas
Clinical Professor
The Ohio State University Medical Center
Columbus, Ohio

AnnMarie Liapakis, MD (Chapter 3)
Fellow, Division of Gasteroneterology and
Hepatology
New York Presbyterian Weill Cornell Medical
Center
New York, New York

Michael Ronan Lucey, MD (Chapter 11)
Professor of Medicine
Chief, Division of Gastroenterology and
Hepatology
University of Wisconsin School of Medicine
and Public Health
Madison, Wisconsin

Paul Martin, MD (Chapter 6)
University of Miami
Division of Hepatology
Miami, Florida

Alvaro Martinez-Camacho, MD (Chapter 9)
Fellow, Division of Gastroenterology and
Hepatology
University of Colorado Denver
Aurora, Colorado

Craig J. McClain, MD (Chapter 1)
Associate Vice President for Translational
Research
Departments of Medicine and Pharmacology
& Toxicology
Louisville, Kentucky

Anthony Michaels, MD (Chapter 2)
Assistant Professor of Medicine
The Ohio State University Medical Center
Columbus, Ohio

Arjmand R. Mufti, MD, MRCP (Chapter 8)
Fellow, Department of Gastroenterology
University of Chicago Medical Center
Chicago, Illinois

Kevin D. Mullen, MD (Chapter 16)
MetroHealth Medical Center
Gastroenterology Division
Cleveland, Ohio

Hector Nazario, MD (Chapter 4)
Baylor University Medical Center
Division of Hepatology
Dallas, Texas

Neehar D. Parikh, MD (Chapter 12)
Division of Gastroenterology and Hepatology
Northwestern University Feinberg School of
Medicine
Chicago, Illinois

Robert Perrillo, MD (Chapter 4)
Baylor University Medical Center
Division of Hepatology
Dallas, Texas

Anjana Pillai, MD (Chapter 10)
Assistant Professor of Medicine
Loyola University Medical Center
Maywood, Illinois

Paul J. Pockros, MD (Chapter 5)
Division of Gastroenterology/Hepatology
Scripps Clinic and
Scripps Translational Science Institute
San Diego, California

Fred Poordad, MD (Chapter 7)
Chief, Hepatology
Cedars-Sinai Comprehensive Transplant
Center
Los Angeles, California

Nataliya Razumilava, MD (Chapter 15)
Fellow, Division of Gastroenterology and
Hepatology
Mayo Clinic
Rochester, Minnesota

Nancy Reau, MD (Chapter 8)
Associate Professor of Medicine
University of Chicago Medical Center
Department of Hepatology, Center for Liver
Diseases
Chicago, Illinois

Mary E. Rinella, MD (Chapter 12)
Division of Gastroenterology and
Hepatology
Northwestern University Feinberg School of
Medicine
Chicago, Illinois

Cristina Ripoll, MD (Chapter 13)
Hospital General Universitario Gregorio
Marañón, CIBERehd
Madrid, Spain

Seth N. Sclair, MD (Chapter 6)
Resident, Internal Medicine
Jackson Memorial Hospital
University of Miami Miller School of
Medicine
Miami, Florida

Puneeta Tandon, MD (Chapter 13)
Division of Gastroenterology
University of Alberta
Edmonton, Alberta, Canada

David Hoffman Van Thiel, MD (Chapter 17)
Professor of Medicine/Surgery
Medical Director of Liver Transplantation
Rush University Medical Center
Chicago, Illinois

Lisa VanWagner, MD (Chapter 12)
Fellow, Division of Gastroenterology and
Hepatology
Northwestern University
Chicago, Illinois

Julia Wattacheril, MD, MPH (Chapter 3)
Transplant Hepatology fellow
Columbia University Medical Center
New York, New York

Jeffrey Weissman, MD (Chapter 5)
Division of Gastroenterology/Hepatology
Scripps Clinic
San Diego, California

Preface

The field of hepatology is full of controversies and clinical dilemmas. We face them every day as we manage our patients and do our best to use evidence-based medicine to assist us in making correct choices. Most controversies do not lend themselves to easy decisions even when we have all of the available medical information and the latest literature findings at our disposal. These clinical conundrums are a test of our diagnostic and therapeutic skills, but are useful in pushing our field ahead by identifying areas of uncertainty. We all know what these controversies are, and have debated them amongst our colleagues. You may have wondered what the true experts do when faced with the same dilemmas. This book is an attempt to crawl into the minds of the experts as they weigh the evidence for and against 17 controversial areas in hepatology.

Controversies in Hepatology was developed based upon the principle of an academic debate. Each expert could solicit 2 fellow trainees (or junior colleagues) to present an evidenced-based argument for and against (pro and con) each statement. The expert would then summarize the key points of each argument and develop a concluding statement. I have been impressed, as I hope you will be, by the rigor with which each argument was developed and crafted by the trainees and junior colleagues. While reading these, I was occasionally left wondering how the experts would choose a final solution, since each argument was so persuasive.

In preparing this book, I have attempted to select topics that were timely and the references as current as possible. Nonetheless, these are moving targets. What are controversies today will hopefully be resolved in the future. Yet some stay with us for many years and seem almost intractable as new research adds new subtleties to the controversy. Often these persistent debates tend to be more ethical dilemmas than scientific misunderstandings, but both deserve our attention and thoughtful dialogue.

In this book, I have divided the chapters into the following sections: Acute Liver Disease, Chronic Hepatitis B and C, Liver Tumors, and Other Chronic Liver Diseases and Cirrhosis. I have selected "experts" as much for their clinical and teaching skills as for their academic contributions to the field. Furthermore, the authors and their junior colleagues were under a fairly severe time constraint so that the published results would be as relevant as possible. They have succeeded admirably.

Who is this book written for? Clearly, hepatologists and their trainees will find the arguments to be a good starting point for further discussion and may even stimulate research initiatives in a particular area. General gastroenterologists will appreciate the succinct development of each topic and the helpful tables and "key points" to rapidly review the controversies in their day-to-day practice. Primary care physicians may also find this book to be a useful addition to their library, remembering that chronic liver disease and liver cancer is one of the top ten causes of death in men over fifty years of age. Finally, medical educators will find that the evidenced-based arguments represent an excellent model to teach future doctors the important skills required in weighing evidence and arriving at an outcome.

I hope you agree with me that *Controversies in Hepatology: The Experts Analyze Both Sides* is both a thoughtful and fun read that will stimulate you in a unique and provocative way.

Foreword

We as hepatologists surely have our share of controversies and dilemmas. There is no doubt that vigorous discussion stimulates thinking and forces further consideration of the implications of the decisions we make. The innovative physician gains from expert reviews and assessment of effective evidence-based approaches. When we are not certain what we should do, we do what we know (or think we know) until more definitive and persuasive information becomes available. Hepatologists—both established and those new to our specialty—will gain from reading the thoughtful, concise discussions presented in *Controversies in Hepatology*.

The editor and the authors of *Controversies in Hepatology: The Experts Analyze Both Sides* are to be congratulated on the choice of topics that are presented. These are timely and topical issues; most hepatologists will immediately recall discussions about each. The seventeen issues are well chosen and the experts who debate them have considerable experience and established credentials. Focused and pertinent documentation supporting the various opinions gives us a glimpse of where we have made progress and, equally important, identifies areas for which we need refined or even novel approaches. The book is well edited, and there is a reassuring consistency in the quality of the presentations.

Many of the decisions we make in our practices of hepatology have momentous consequences. We all have faced the decision regarding when (or if) to proceed to resection of a presumed or proven benign hepatic mass. Furthermore, there are ongoing debates as to whether patients who are actively drinking and have alcohol-induced cirrhosis should undergo a prolonged (often 6 months) abstinence period before being considered a candidate for liver transplant. Surely the role of corticosteroid therapy in the treatment of patients with severe alcoholic hepatitis remains a topic often and vigorously discussed. The choices of therapeutic approaches in patients who have primary sclerosing cholangitis, autoimmune hepatitis, and hepatic encephalopathy continue to be discussed. Underlying the difficulties in many situations is the recognition that there are no clear therapeutic winners for much of what we encounter. And then there are the issues concerning the treatment of chronic hepatitis B and chronic hepatitis C. The advances in treatment options for chronic viral hepatitis have been spectacular and, of course, the new approaches for treating hepatitis viruses are now on the verge of expansion. This will initiate a new phase of issues, expectations, and opportunities. *Controversies in Hepatology* helps define and frame a variety of these issues. I thoroughly enjoyed reading the volume and look forward to the next edition to see which dilemmas have receded and what new issues have come to the fore.

Willis C. Maddrey, MD
Professor of Internal Medicine
UT Southwestern Medical Center
Dallas, Texas

SECTION I
ACUTE LIVER DISEASE

ALCOHOLIC HEPATITIS
PENTOXIFYLLINE VERSUS STEROIDS

Leila Gobejishvili, PhD; Neil Crittenden, MD; and Craig J. McClain, MD

Alcoholic liver disease (ALD) remains a leading cause of death from liver disease in the United States and worldwide. In studies from the Veterans Administration, patients with cirrhosis and superimposed alcoholic hepatitis (AH) had a greater than 60% mortality over a 4-year period of time, with a large portion of those deaths occurring in the first month.[1] Thus, the prognosis for this disease is more ominous than for many common types of cancer such as breast, prostate, and colon. Unfortunately, there is still no Federal Drug Administration (FDA)-approved or universally accepted drug therapy for any stage of ALD. Two drugs, pentoxifylline (PTX) and steroids, are often used "off label" to treat AH, and competing arguments are made for their use.

POINT

Pentoxifylline/Phosphodiesterase Inhibitors: Potential Mechanisms of Action in Alcoholic Hepatitis

by Leila Gobejishvili, PhD

Inflammatory cytokines, particularly TNF, play a significant role in the pathogenesis of liver injury and the clinical/biochemical abnormalities of AH.[2] The authors of this chapter and others have reported increased serum levels of TNF, increased monocyte TNF production, and hepatic immunohistochemical staining for TNF in AH that frequently correlate with disease severity and mortality.[2-4] Patients with AH commonly have endotoxemia,[5] which activates the oxidative stress–sensitive transcription factor NFκB, thus modulating the synthesis of several adhesion molecules and inflammatory cytokines, including TNF.[6]

An important role for anti-inflammatory cytokines, particularly IL-10, is increasingly recognized in the pathogenesis of ALD.[7] IL-10 is a critical anti-inflammatory cytokine, suppressing

Jensen D.
Controversies in Hepatology: The Experts Analyze Both
Sides (pp 3-10)
© 2011 SLACK Incorporated

both immunoproliferative and inflammatory responses.[8] Indeed, depressed monocyte synthesis of IL-10 has been reported to play a role in increased TNF production and subsequent liver injury in ALD.[9] In addition, IL-10 may also exert antifibrotic effects in the liver through mechanisms such as inhibition of collagen gene transcription and increased collagenase expression by hepatic stellate cells.[10]

PTX is a nonselective phosphodiesterase (PDE) inhibitor. Cyclic nucleotide PDE are ubiquitously present in different tissues and cells. Their function is to hydrolyze adenosine 3′, 5′-cyclic monophosphate (cAMP) and guanosine 3′, 5′-cyclic monophosphate (cGMP) and maintain the homeostasis of these important second messengers. PDE consists of 11 different gene families (PDE1 through PDE11), each of which includes more than one distinct gene. PTX treatment increases intracellular concentrations of cAMP and cGMP. Increased cAMP has been shown to positively modulate the cytokine inflammatory response, with a decrease in the proinflammatory cytokine, TNF, and an increase in the anti-inflammatory cytokine, IL-10.

Although the critical role of TNF in the progression of ALD is well established, the mechanism(s) by which ethanol enhances TNF expression, particularly in monocytes/macrophages, is still being defined. The authors evaluated the effect of increased cellular cAMP levels on lipopolysaccharide (LPS)-inducible TNF expression in monocytes/macrophages exposed chronically to ethanol using a nondegradable, cell-permeable cAMP analogue (dbcAMP). Chronic ethanol exposure resulted in a decline in basal and stimulatable cAMP levels, and increasing cellular cAMP levels led to the inhibition of the synergistic enhancement in TNF-α expression caused by ethanol and LPS. Consistent with our in vitro findings, Kupffer cells obtained from a clinically relevant enteral alcohol feeding model of ALD also showed decreased intracellular cAMP levels and increased expression of TNF compared to Kupffer cells from pair-fed rats.[11]

Agents that enhance cAMP (such as dbcAMP and the PDE4 specific inhibitor, Rolipram) have been used in in vivo studies to protect against LPS- and alcohol-induced hepatitis.[12,13] These studies clearly showed that increased cAMP levels inhibited TNF-α production from activated macrophages/Kupffer cells, and partially protected the liver from the injury. Furthermore, cAMP treatment ameliorated the increase of liver fat storage and changes in the fatty acid composition in the livers of ethanol-fed animals, and the ethanol-induced increase in CYP2E1 protein was partially inhibited by cAMP treatment.[13] The critical role of PDE4B in LPS-induced TNF expression has been extensively studied by Conti's laboratory.[14] Using PDE4B-deficient mice, they demonstrated that PDE4B gene activation by LPS is essential for LPS-activated TNF responses and ablation of PDE4B gene protected mice from LPS-induced shock.

Importantly, we have shown that chronic ethanol exposure increases LPS-inducible expression of PDE4B in monocytes/macrophages of both human and murine origin, and this is associated with enhanced NFB activation and transcriptional activity and subsequent priming of monocytes/ macrophages leading to enhanced LPS-inducible TNF-production.[15] Thus, there is substantial experimental data supporting the rationale for PDE inhibition and increasing cAMP in the treatment of AH using PTX (or possibly more specific inhibitors).

Pentoxifylline Therapy in Alcoholic Hepatitis

Akriviadis et al[16] in a prospective, randomized, double-blind clinical trial evaluated the effects of PTX in severe AH (DF ≥32). Forty-nine patients received 400 mg of PTX orally 3 times daily and 52 received placebo for 4 weeks. Primary outcome variables were survival and development of hepatorenal syndrome (HRS). PTX treatment significantly improved survival; 12 (24.5%) PTX patients died as compared to 24 (46%) placebo patients ($P = 0.037$; relative risk = 0.59). PTX also decreased HRS as a cause of death; 6 (50%) PTX-treated patients died of renal failure compared with 22 (92%) dead control patients. A second study from India compared PTX to prednisone in a 28 day randomized, double-blind, controlled study (which ultimately converted to an open-label protocol for 2 additional months).[17] The PTX group showed a significant survival benefit at 3 months; of 34 patients receiving PTX, 5 patients died as compared to 12 deaths in a series of 34 patients receiving prednisolone. Similarly, PTX was associated with a lower model for end-stage liver disease (MELD) score at 28 days, and a greater renal protective effect was noted. While these studies show beneficial effects of PTX versus placebo and prednisolone, a third study showed no beneficial effects in switching from prednisolone to PTX, if steroid therapy failure was noted at 1 week (steroid-resistant patients).[18]

KEY POINTS

- Two randomized trials support use of PTX (400 mg tid) in severe AH.
- PTX is renal protective and decreases hepatorenal syndrome.
- PTX has both anti-inflammatory and anti-fibrotic properties and has potential for long-term use.
- A switch from steroids to PTX in steroid-resistant patients is not effective.

COUNTERPOINT

Mechanisms of Action in Alcoholic Hepatitis

by Neil Crittenden, MD

Corticosteroids are a subclass of glucocorticoids, endogenously produced hormones with known anti-inflammatory and immunosuppressive properties. This class of drugs has been successfully used to treat a wide variety of chronic inflammatory diseases, and their mechanism of action on cells such as Kupffer cells, monocytes, and endothelial cells has been extensively investigated. Glucocorticoids can both suppress and activate multiple pro- and anti-inflammatory genes, as well as exert post-transcriptional effects.[19-21] Glucocorticoids transverse the plasma membrane and bind to glucocorticoid receptors (GR) in the cytoplasm. Following ligand binding, activated GRs are released from chaperone proteins (eg, heat shock protein 90) and translocate to the nucleus. There, the GR homodimerize and bind to the glucocorticoid response elements (GREs) in the promoter region of glucocorticoid responsive genes to switch them either on or off. Glucocorticoids inhibit production of several key inflammatory molecules thought to play a role in AH by inhibiting transcription factors such as NFκB and AP1.[19] This inhibition is modulated in a large part by recruitment of histone deacetylase-2 (HDAC2) to the activated inflammatory gene by the GR. Glucocorticoids can also have post-transcriptional effects on certain cytokines, especially TNF-α, which has an unstable mRNA that is rapidly degraded by RNAases but stabilized by certain inflammatory mediators. Glucocorticoids can inhibit this stabilization process and result in more rapid degradation of mRNA (thus inhibiting proinflammatory cytokine production).

Importantly, there is a subset of patients that are glucocorticoid resistant (usually about 30%). This glucocorticoid resistance can be due to multiple mechanisms; reduced HDAC2 activity expression occurs in some patients who respond poorly.[19,20] Oxidative and nitrosative stress (seen in AH) can inhibit HDAC2 activity. Macrophage migration inhibitory factor (MIF) is a proinflammatory cytokine that has antiglucocorticoid effects.[22] Lastly, levels of GRβ, an alternatively-spliced form of GR that essentially acts as a dominant negative inhibitor of glucocorticoid action, is increased in some steroid-resistant disease states.[19-21] Thus, our knowledge of mechanisms of glucocorticoid action and resistance has been markedly expanded. This may play an important role in steroid therapy in AH and potentially provide mechanisms to enhance steroid effectiveness in patients who demonstrate early (1 week) failure to respond to steroids.

Corticosteroid Therapy in Alcoholic Hepatitis

Corticosteroids have been used for 5 decades in the treatment of AH with improving results due to enhanced patient selection. Maddrey et al first highlighted factors associated with poor prognosis in AH and devised the original Maddrey Discriminant Function.[23] Later revised and validated, several trials and meta analyses have consistently shown that patients with a Maddrey's score ≥32 or spontaneous hepatic encephalopathy treated with steroids have a statistically significant reduction in mortality compared to placebo.[24,25] In one of these analyses, it was estimated the number of patients needed to treat with corticosteroids to prevent one death was 5[24] (see Table 1-1).

The recognition that select patients benefit, while others termed *nonresponders* are at increased risk for side effects without apparent advantage, has led researchers to establish other early clinical predictors of steroid responsiveness. The Early Change in Bilirubin Level (ECBL) determines whether bilirubin level at 7 days is lower than the bilirubin level on the first day of treatment, and it is one tool to identify corticosteroid responders.[26] The subsequent Lille Model also allows patients to receive a 7-day course of corticosteroids and it judges the responsiveness based on an algorithm combining age, renal insufficiency, albumin, prothrombin time, bilirubin, and evolution of bilirubin on the last day.[27] Patients with a score of greater than 0.45 had a poor 6-month survival rate (25%) and could be discontinued from corticosteroids. However, those patients with scores less than the cutoff of 0.45 had an 85% survival rate and would benefit from continued corticosteroid treatment. The model was based on 295 patients with severe AH with a discriminate function ≥32 or encephalopathy and the model was subsequently validated prospectively in 118 more patients.

Although infection has been classically viewed as a contraindication to corticosteroids, a study using the Lille Model found that being a responder to corticosteroids was independently associated with survival ($P = 0.000001$) while an infection was not ($P = 0.52$). The authors urged that infection should not been a contraindication to corticosteroids.[28]

Table 1-1.
PROGNOSTIC SCORING SYSTEMS IN ALCOHOLIC HEPATITIS
Maddrey Discriminant Function (DF) = 4.6 x (patient PT − control PT) + Total Bilirubin (mg/dl) Poor prognosis >32 Example: 4.6 x (18-12)+ 12 = 39.6
Other examples of scoring systems include MELD, Glasgow Score, Lille Model, etc.[30,31] All calculators are available online.

Recent experiments have further investigated steroid unresponsiveness, and a new assay is being developed to predict responsiveness sooner. Lymphocytes from acute AH patients were treated with increasing concentrations of dexamethasone ex vivo. The maximum inhibition of lymphocyte proliferation (Imax) was measured, and dexamethasone impaired growth in control patients (Imax = 95%) more than AH patients (Imax = 67%, P = 0.0002). In AH, steroid-responsive patients with an ECBL had a higher mean Imax (74%) compared to patients without an ECBL (58%, P <0.05). Imax was also used as a marker of recovery. In 7 patients at follow-up, mean Imax was higher (92%) than at presentation (70%, P = 0.01). The assay can predict steroid responsiveness at day 4 or earlier, helping to minimize steroid-related complications.[29] Moreover, ex vivo treatment of AH lymphocytes with theophylline (enhance HDAC recruitment) improved steroid responsiveness.[29]

Current class I, level A guidelines from both the American College of Gastroenterology (ACG) and the American Association for the Study of Liver Diseases (AASLD) advise that patients with severe AH with a discriminate function ≥32 and lacking contradiction to steroids should be considered for a 4-week course of prednisolone 40 mg daily followed by a taper.[30,31]

KEY POINTS

- Meta-analyses support use of corticosteroids in severe AH without contraindications (40 mg/day).
- Use early change in bilirubin level (1 week) to monitor clinical response.
- ~30% of patients with many inflammatory processes including AH are steroid resistant.
- Unclear if steroid unresponsive AH can be medically converted to responsive.

EXPERT OPINION

Conclusions

Craig J. McClain, MD

This is less of a heated debate and more of a "feel-good" summary. The literature suggests that steroids are generally first-line therapy for AH in patients who do not have contraindications, such as gastrointestinal (GI) bleeding. As an initial steroid skeptic, my enthusiasm has increased somewhat because of the early change in bilirubin level data.[26] Thus, we now have "steroid-stopping rules" analogous to stopping rules for hepatitis C therapy. Importantly, about one-third of patients are nonresponders to steroids. A major question is: are these nonresponders too sick to respond to any treatment or are they metabolically steroid nonresponders who might be converted to responder status with medical therapy? This concept is under active investigation in the pulmonary field.[19-21] This concept has also received initial evaluation in AH, using theophylline ex vivo as an HDAC modulator.[29] Another "steroid-sensitizing strategy" would be blocking MIF activity, a cytokine that inhibits corticosteroid effects.[22] Steroids also have the treatment advantage of being available in intravenous form for patients unable to take oral medications, such as severely encephalopathic AH subjects.

Substantial insight into phosphodiesterases (PDEs) and the role of cAMP in experimental liver disease and cytokine metabolism has occurred over the past decade.[11-15] PTX is a nonspecific PDE inhibitor. More specific PDE4 inhibitors are being developed and are in clinical trials for pulmonary disease, where steroid resistance has been studied extensively. A major side effect of PDE4 inhibition is nausea that is induced when the drug crosses the blood-brain barrier. Our research team is taking the experimental approach of targeting PDE4 inhibitor therapy to the liver (via liposomes), which may allow greater drug delivery to the target organ with less toxicity. The good news is that there are now 2 studies showing the beneficial effects of PTX in AH and documenting great efficacy in preventing HRS. We regularly use PTX in AH patients with marginal renal function (creatinine >1.1/1.2 mg/dL).[16,17] We tend to use PTX as our first-line therapy in most patients, and we often continue this for prolonged periods of time, as this is a highly safe drug that may have long-term antifibrotic properties. We do use steroids first line in some patients who have severe AH with prominent leukocytosis, neutrophilia, and fever, and we use steroids when AH patients cannot tolerate oral medications. While a switch from steroids to PTX in steroid nonresponders does not appear to be beneficial, a large multicenter study from France has just been completed evaluating potential efficacy of initial combination therapy of PTX in addition to steroids as compared to steroids alone. We should have the results of this study in the near future, and in the interim there would seem to be no contraindications to this dual approach.

Summary

We are fortunate to have 2 drugs with some efficacy for AH. Our initial approach is different from the ACG and the AASLD guidelines in that we usually utilize PTX as first-line therapy. Physicians now have important new information concerning steroid responsiveness in AH, new insight into the role of PDEs in AH, and better understanding of the best way to employ these approaches in AH. Thus, the future is bright for even more improved therapy for this highly morbid disease process in the near future.

References

1. Chedid A, Mendenhall CL, Gartside P, et al. Prognostic factors in alcoholic liver disease. VA Cooperative Study Group. *Am J Gastroenterol.* 1991;86:210-216.
2. McClain CJ, Cohen DA. Increased tumor necrosis factor production by monocytes in alcoholic hepatitis. *Hepatology.* 1989;9:349-351.
3. Bird GL, Sheron N, Goka AK, et al. Increased plasma tumor necrosis factor in severe alcoholic hepatitis. *Ann Intern Med.* 1990;112:917-920.
4. Felver ME, Mezey E, McGuire M, et al. Plasma tumor necrosis factor alpha predicts decreased long-term survival in severe alcoholic hepatitis. *Alcohol Clin Exp Res.* 1990;14:255-259.
5. Bode JC, Parlesak A, Bode C. Gut derived bacterial toxins (endotoxin) and alcohol liver disease. In: Agarwal P, Seitz HK, eds. *Alcohol in Health and Disease.* New York, NY: Marcel Dekker; 2001:369-386.
6. Muller JM, Ziegler-Heitbrock HW, et al. Nuclear factor kappa B, a mediator of lipopolysaccharide effects. *Immunobiology.* 1993;187:233-256.
7. Hill DB, D'Souza NB, Lee EY, et al. A role for interleukin-10 in alcohol induced liver sensitization to bacterial lipopolysaccharide. *Alcohol Clin Exp Res.* 2002;26(1):74-82.
8. Moore KW, O'Garra AO, de Waal Malefyt R, et al. Interleukin-10. *Ann Rev Immunol.* 1993;11:165-190.
9. Le Moine O, Marchant A, De Groote D, et al. Role of defective monocyte interleukin-10 release in tumor necrosis factor-alpha overproduction in alcoholic cirrhosis. *Hepatology.* 1995;22:1436-1439.
10. Wang SC, Ohata M, Scrum L, et al. Expression of interleukin-10 by in vitro and in vivo activated hepatic stellate cells. *J Biol Chem.* 1998;273:302-308.

11. Gobejishvili L, Barve S, Joshi-Barve S, et al. Chronic ethanol mediated decrease in cellular cAMP leads to enhanced LPS-inducible NFkB activity and TNF expression in macrophages: relevance to alcoholic liver disease. *Am J Physiol Gastrointest Liver Physiol.* 2006;291:G681-G688.

12. Taguchi I, Oka K, Kitamura K, et al. Protection by a cyclic AMP-specific phosphodiesterase inhibitor, rolipram, and dibutyryl cyclic AMP against Propionibacterium acnes and lipopolysaccharide-induced mouse hepatitis. *Inflamm Res.* 1999;48(7):380-385.

13. Gouillon ZQ, Miyamoto K, Donohue TM, et al. Role of CYP2E1 in the pathogenesis of alcoholic liver disease: modifications by cAMP and ubiquitin-proteasome pathway. *Front Biosci.* 1999;4:A16-A25.

14. Jin SL, Lan L, Zoudilova M, et al. Specific role of phosphodiesterase 4B in lipopolysaccharide-induced signaling in mouse macrophages. *J Immunology.* 2005;175:1523-1531.

15. Gobejishvili L, Barve S, Joshi-Barve S, et al. Enhanced PDE4B expression augments LPS-inducible TNF expression in ethanol-primed monocytes: relevance to alcoholic liver disease. *Am J Physiol Gastrointest Liver Physiol.* 2008;295:718-724.

16. Akriviadis E, Botla R, Briggs W, et al. Pentoxifylline improves short-term survival in severe acute alcoholic hepatitis: a double-blind, placebo-controlled trial. *Gastroenterology.* 2000;119(6):1637-1648.

17. De BK, Gangopadhyay S, Dutta D, et al. Pentoxifylline versus prednisolone for severe alcoholic hepatitis: a randomized controlled trial. *World J Gastroenterol.* 2009;15(1):1613-1619.

18. Louvet A, Diaz E, Dharancy S, et al. Early switch to pentoxifylline in patients with severe alcoholic hepatitis is inefficient in non-responders to corticosteroids. *J Hepatol.* 48(3):465-470.

19. Barnes, PJ. Mechanisms and resistance in glucocorticoid control of inflammation. *J Steroid Biochem Mol Biol.* 2010;120:76-85.

20. Rajendrasozhan S, Yang SR, Edirisinghe I, et al. Deacetylases and NF-kappaB in redox regulation of cigarette smoke-induced lung inflammation: epigenetics in pathogenesis of COPD. *Antioxid Redox Signal.* 2008;10(4):799-811.

21. Rogatsky I, Ivashkiv LB. Glucocorticoid modulation of cytokine signaling. *Tissue Antigens.* 2006;68(1):1-12.

22. Van Molle W, Libert C. How glucocorticoids control their own strength and the balance between pro- and anti-inflammatory mediators. *Eur J Immunol.* 2005;35(12):3396-3399.

23. Maddrey WC, Boitnott JK, Bedine MS, et al. Corticosteroid therapy of alcoholic hepatitis. *Gastroenterology.* 1978;75:193-199.

24. Mathurin P, Mendenhall CL, Carithers RL, et al. Corticosteroids improve short-term survival in patients with severe alcoholic hepatitis (AH): individual data analysis of the last three randomized placebo controlled double blind trials of corticosteroids in severe AH. *J Hepatol.* 2002;36:480-487.

25. Rambaldi A, Saconato HH, Christensen E, et al. Systematic review: glucocorticosteroids for alcoholic hepatitis--a Cochrane Hepato-Biliary Group systematic review with meta-analyses and trial sequential analyses of randomized clinical trials. *Aliment Pharmacol Ther.* 2008;27:1167-1178.

26. Mathurin P, Abdelnour M, Ramond MJ, et al. Early change in bilirubin levels is an important prognostic factor in severe alcoholic hepatitis treated with prednisolone. *Hepatology.* 2003;38:1363-1369.

27. Louvet A, Naveau S, Abdelnour M, et al. The Lille model: a new tool for therapeutic strategy in patients with severe alcoholic hepatitis treated with steroids. *Hepatology.* 2007;45:1348-1354.

28. Louvet A, Wartel F, Castel H, et al. Infection in patients with severe alcoholic hepatitis treated with steroids: early response to therapy is the key factor. *Gastroenterology.* 2009;137:541-548.

29. Kendrick SF, Henderson E, Palmer J, et al. Theophylline improves steroid sensitivity in acute alcoholic hepatitis. *Hepatology.* 2010;52:126-131.

30. O'Shea RS, Dasarathy S, McCullough AJ. Alcoholic liver disease. *Am J Gastroenterol.* 2010;105:14-32.

31. O'Shea RS, Dasarathy S, McCullough AJ. Alcoholic liver disease. *Hepatology.* 2010;51:307-328.

IS N-ACETYLCYSTEINE EFFECTIVE IN ALL CASES OF NON-ACETAMINOPHEN ACUTE LIVER FAILURE?

A. James Hanje, MD; Anthony Michaels, MD; and William M. Lee, MD

N-acetylcysteine (NAC) is a highly effective antidote for acetaminophen-induced liver injury and can protect patients against very large doses of this highly toxic agent. It was natural that clinicians impressed by the drug would seek other uses for it. It has been thought to have possible benefit in protecting against renal tubular cell injury following radiocontrast and possibly other situations such as gram-negative sepsis, but the natural situation to try it in is acute liver failure not due to acetaminophen. Several small or uncontrolled trials led to the Acute Liver Failure Study Group mounting a placebo-controlled, double-blind trial in 1999 that was concluded in 2006 and published in 2009. Benefit was shown in subgroups and the results have remained somewhat controversial. Here, we play out that controversy and will let the reader decide what the appropriate course of action should be next time a patient with severe liver injury shows up in your emergency department.

POINT

N-Acetylcysteine for All Non-Acetaminophen Acute Liver Failure

by A. James Hanje, MD

NAC has been shown to reduce or prevent liver damage in acetaminophen overdose.[1] However, its role in non-acetaminophen acute liver failure (ALF) has not been studied until recently. Few trials have been performed to date. Nonetheless, the possible beneficial role for NAC in non-acetaminophen ALF is intriguing given the lack of alternative, established treatments other than liver transplantation for this patient population.

Many mechanisms have been proposed to explain the ability of NAC to minimize liver damage in ALF. In acetaminophen toxicity, one of the primary protective mechanisms of NAC involves replenishing glutathione stores. In non-acetaminophen ALF, however, glutathione depletion is not thought to be a primary contributor to hepatic necrosis. In a small study of both acetaminophen and non-acetaminophen ALF, an increase in oxygen delivery and consumption was observed in both groups with NAC. This appeared to be due primarily to an increase in cardiac output and mean arterial pressure in patients receiving NAC, despite a fall in systemic vascular resistance.[2]

NAC was studied in retrospective fashion in 170 children with non-acetaminophen ALF between 1989 and 2004.[3] Although similar percentages of patients were admitted to the ICU (71% in group 1 as compared to 77% in group 2, P = ns), outcomes differed significantly between the 2 groups, with length of stay, 10 year actuarial survival, and survival without transplant all showing significant benefit in the NAC-treated group. Of interest, 8 children (10.8%) experienced adverse events while receiving intravenous NAC, with only one case of bronchospasm reported. Although limited by its retrospective design, this large clinical trial demonstrated compelling evidence for improved clinical outcomes in this setting.

In the largest clinical trial to date, the Acute Liver Failure Study Group reported the use of NAC in non-acetaminophen ALF in adult patients.[4] Composed of 24 liver transplant centers throughout the United States, the group enrolled 173 patients with non-acetaminophen ALF between 1998 and 2006. Using a prospective, randomized, placebo-controlled design, the investigators assigned 81 patients to receive intravenous NAC and 92 patients to receive placebo for 72 hours. The primary endpoint was survival at 3 weeks, with secondary endpoints including transplant-free survival and transplant rate.

Patient characteristics between the placebo and treatment groups were similar in terms of coma grade I through II on admission—62% and 73%, respectively—despite over-representation of this group within the study cohort (114 patients [66%] were coma grade I or II, while 59 patients [35%] were coma grade III or IV). While overall survival between the treatment and placebo group was not different at 21 days—70% versus 66%, respectively (P = 0.283)— transplant-free survival was significantly higher in the treatment group than in the placebo group (40% versus 27%, P = .043). Figure 2-1 shows the data from the ALFSG trial depicted

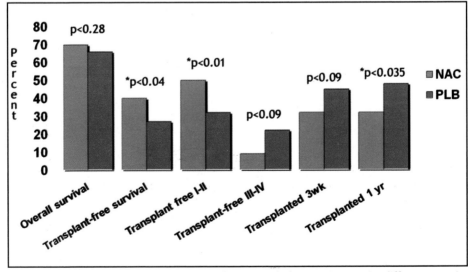

Figure 2-1. Primary/secondary outcomes in the NAC trial. The most impressive difference was in transplant-free survival in coma grades I-II.   * = statistically significant

Table 2-1.				
NAC RESULTS BY ETIOLOGY				
OVERALL SURVIVAL / TRANSPLANT-FREE SURVIVAL				
DILI n=45	17/26 65%	15/19 79%	7/26 27%	11/19 58%
AIH n=26	10/15 67%	7/11 64%	4/15 27%	1/11 9%
HBV n=37	6/12 50%	19/25 76%	2/12 17%	10/25 40%
Indeterm n=41	18/26 69%	9/15 60%	6/26 23%	6/15 40%

as bar graphs, showing data for the stratification groups to highlight the differences between overall and spontaneous survival. When broken down by coma grade, the benefit of NAC appeared confined only to those patients with grade I to II coma. Transplant-free survival in patients who received NAC was 52% as compared to 30% for those who received placebo (P = .010). In patients with grade III to IV coma, transplant-free survival in the NAC group was only 9% as compared to 22% in the placebo group (P = .912). Although the transplant rate was lower in the NAC group (32%), this was not statistically significant when compared to the placebo group (45%, P = .093). The etiology of ALF for the majority of patients fell into 4 categories: drug-induced liver injury (DILI), autoimmune hepatitis, hepatitis B (HBV) and indeterminate (Table 2-1). Benefit seemed greatest for the DILI and hepatitis B groups. Safety and tolerability of intravenous NAC was similar to placebo except for increased reports of nausea and vomiting (14% versus 4%, P = .031). Only one case of bronchospasm was reported. The authors concluded from this study that intravenous NAC administration improved transplant-free survival in patients with coma grade I to II non-acetaminophen ALF, while patients with coma grade III to IV did not benefit and typically required emergency liver transplantation.

Summary

There is accumulating evidence from several trials, albeit not perfect ones, to suggest potential benefit to the use of intravenous NAC in non-acetaminophen ALF. It is true that there are few studies assessing clinical endpoints, and only one has been prospectively designed and randomized. ALF is an extremely rare condition and non-acetaminophen ALF comprises less than 50% of patients.[5] The Acute Liver Failure Study Group took over 8 years to complete their prospectively designed, randomized trial. It appeared to be adequately powered. But the critical condition of the patients involved, the rapid progression of disease, and taking into consideration the need to simultaneously evaluate for urgent liver transplantation makes the rigorous study of this condition extremely challenging. The conclusions obtained to date should be recognized as promising, and highlight the need for future, collaborative, multicenter studies to assess clinical outcomes.

KEY POINTS

■ Improved transplant-free survival was observed for non-acetaminophen ALF patients treated with IV NAC in a carefully controlled trial.

■ Benefit was confined to early coma grade (I to II) patients.

■ Further investigation into the use of IV NAC for non-acetaminophen ALF is needed.

COUNTERPOINT

N-Acetylcysteine Has Not Been Shown to Be Effective for All Non-Acetaminophen Acute Liver Failure

by Anthony Michaels, MD

There have been few studies published evaluating the role of N-acetylcysteine (NAC) in the treatment of non-acetaminophen acute liver failure (ALF). As noted previously, glutathione depletion is not thought to be involved in the pathogenesis of non-acetaminophen-induced ALF.[6] Early studies looking at the use of NAC in non-acetaminophen ALF were smaller studies that did not adequately assess clinical outcomes.[6,7] The pediatric study by Kortsalioudaki et al[3] did demonstrate a shorter length of hospital stay and had a greater overall survival, which included survival with the native liver and after liver transplantation with NAC, but there were no significant differences found between the 2 groups in lengths of intensive care stay, incidences of death without liver transplantation, numbers of transplants required, and rates of retransplantation. Since the study was retrospective and the 2 treatment groups were sequential with the control group treated during the earlier time period, factors other than NAC may have affected the outcomes, such as improvement in overall intensive care during the later study period, not just the addition of NAC. For example, a statistically significantly higher percentage of inotropic support occurred within the NAC treatment group. As the authors highlighted, this likely indicates a more aggressive intensive care treatment strategy in the management of their disease.[3] Changes to intensive care unit protocols and more proactive management strategies that occur over decades alter patient survival and the ultimate outcome.

Similar data were also reported in an adult population in Pakistan, evaluating the role of NAC in non-acetaminophen ALF.[8] In this study, patients treated with NAC had decreased mortality and improved survival with their native liver compared to patients that were not treated with NAC. The virtue (and vice) in countries where transplant is not available is that the "true" outcome is known and no transplant rescue can occur. However, similar to the study by Kortsalioudaki et al, the 2 groups being compared were not treated at the same point in time. Again, the patients not treated with NAC were collected retrospectively from 2000 to 2003, while the NAC patients were from 2004 to 2007 and prospectively enrolled. In addition, the 2 treatment groups differed in a number of categories: the NAC treatment group were significantly younger, had more significant features of raised intracranial pressure, required mechanical ventilation more often, and had significantly higher bilirubin levels at the time of admission.

These discrepancies make it difficult to compare the treatment groups and to conclude if NAC is truly beneficial in this patient population. Even though these studies reported a survival benefit of NAC, they still have flaws.

In the Acute Liver Failure Study Group (ALFSG) NAC trial, 92 patients with non-acetaminophen ALF were randomized to receive placebo, while 81 patients were randomized to the NAC treatment group. The primary outcomes were not met: overall 3-week survival ($P = 0.283$) and transplantation rates ($P = 0.093$) did not significantly differ between the 2 treatment groups, and treatment with NAC did not significantly shorten hospital admissions compared with the placebo group.[4] The 2 study groups were similar except the placebo group had significantly more females and longer median duration between jaundice and encephalopathy compared to NAC treatment group and the study was blinded, controlled, and prospective. The NAC treatment group was found to have had a significantly higher transplant-free survival rate than the placebo group ($P = 0.043$). However, when the transplant-free survival data was further analyzed, only patients with coma grades I to II in the NAC treatment group had a significantly higher transplant-free survival rate at 3 weeks and 1 year. Patients with coma grades III to IV in the NAC treatment group actually did not have a significant difference in transplant-free survival when compared to the coma III to IV patients in the placebo group ($P = 0.912$). Odds ratio analysis was performed comparing the 2 treatment groups and actually showed an odds ratio (0.33) favoring the placebo group for transplant-free survival at 3 weeks who presented with more of an advanced coma grade of III to IV.

Summary

Only a few studies have been performed analyzing the clinical benefit of NAC in patients with non-acetaminophen ALF, and only one of these studies was prospective and randomized. Even though patients with early encephalopathy with non-acetaminophen ALF may benefit from NAC, the greatest impact on survival in this patient population remains liver transplantation. Therefore, early referral and establishment at a transplant center remains the gold standard in the management of this patient population.

KEY POINTS

- Few studies have evaluated NAC for non-acetaminophen ALF; only one controlled trial has been performed.
- NAC demonstrated no benefit for non-acetaminophen ALF presenting with advanced stages of coma.
- The greatest impact on survival in this population is liver transplantation.

N-Acetylcysteine Appears to Be an Effective Treatment for All Patients With Non-Acetaminophen Acute Liver Failure

by William M. Lee, MD

ALF remains a puzzling and fascinating condition. It begins with multiple etiologies that all produce a similar final result: coma and coagulopathy with a high likelihood of a fatal outcome. Acute liver failure proves—if there was any doubt—the vital role played by the liver in the overall conduct of the body's business. NAC has long been recognized as a highly effective antidote for prevention of acetaminophen toxicity but its use in non-acetaminophen etiologies was only hinted at in the Harrison paper quoted.[2] No firm data were presented to support its use in other forms of ALF. While there have been many attempts at therapy for the overall condition of acute liver failure, only NAC has borne fruit, to date. Circumstantial evidence supports its efficacy in other settings such as renal tubular necrosis due to radio-contrast. Studies in acute liver failure have been flawed because of either limited patient selection or the study of a single coma grade (grade IV), as seen in the study by the Edinburgh group.[9] The approach taken by the ALF Study Group, funded by the FDA and National Institute of Diabetes and Digestive and Kidney Diseases (NIDDK), was to test in a randomized fashion the efficacy of NAC in the non-acetaminophen setting. The results have been clearly presented already by my colleagues and it is left for me to critique my own study! First, we picked the wrong primary outcome: we initially suggested that spontaneous survival would be the best measure of efficacy but were persuaded that NAC might improve outcomes in transplanted patients as well and so we adopted overall outcome as our primary endpoint. All trials since 1985 in acute liver failure have been compromised by the rescue provided by liver transplantation, which improves survival from an estimated 20% to 28% to nearly 90%. However, the "true" outcome of transplanted patients will never be known; it is presumed to be poor, but not entirely equivalent to death. Despite its inherent flaws, the closest measure of efficacy is spontaneous survival (ie, grouping transplant and death as a common outcome). Nonetheless, we were able to show efficacy of NAC in early coma grades and this makes a great deal of intuitive sense. Outcomes for those reaching advanced coma grades appear to be preordained, occurring largely within 3 days of admission, death, or transplantation; all those eligible in this group will be listed upon arrival at coma grade III. Earlier coma grades reach the 50% outcome point at 10 days, not 3, and thus there is more possibility of improvement in hepatic function and regaining hepatic reserve with milder insults.

Trials in acute liver failure are extremely difficult because of the rarity of the condition, its highly variable outcomes, and the rescue effect of transplantation. Whether improvements in intensive care resulted in improved outcomes remains to be seen. Transplantation is still only available for about 25% of patients with ALF, the remainder either being too sick for transplantation, listed but unable to survive until a graft is available, disqualified for transplantation because of psychosocial reasons, or not sick enough. One main reason for improved survival in recent years has been the increasing numbers of acetaminophen toxicity cases, approaching 50% of all presenting patients, and this group carries a better overall prognosis of about 62% spontaneous survival and 8% transplantation.[5] By contrast, the non-acetaminophen cases carry a 25% spontaneous survival rate, a 40% transplant rate, and 35% death rate in patients who do not receive a graft—still a pretty grim prospect. In our study, it appeared that DILI and hepatitis B (across all coma grades) responded more favorably to NAC than autoimmune hepatitis or indeterminate cases (Table 2-1), but this is speculative since the numbers in each group were quite small.

Summary

NAC appears to benefit those with early stage ALF and offers nothing to those with advanced coma grades, although the studies to date are less than ideal for the reasons cited. NAC is apparently not effective for all patients with non-acetaminophen ALF; only those with some remaining potential for recovery. The most significant benefit was observed in those with drug-induced liver injury or hepatitis B as compared to autoimmune and indeterminate causes. The reasons for these differences are unknown; larger studies would be able to settle these questions but are unlikely to be performed. I predict that the future in this area will involve the use of NAC as a general liver protective or tonic, while more potent anti-inflammatory and proregenerative factors are tested.

References

1. Keays R, Harrison PM, Wendon JA, et al. Intravenous acetylcysteine in paracetamol induced fulminant hepatic failure: a prospective controlled trial. *BMJ.* 1991;303:1024-1029.
2. Harrison PM, Wendon JA, Gimson AE, Alexander GJ, Williams R. Improvement by acetylcysteine of hemodynamics and oxygen transport in fulminant hepatic failure. *N Engl J Med.* 1991;324:1852-1857.
3. Kortsalioudaki C, Taylor RM, Cheeseman P, Bansal S, Mieli-Vergani G, Dhawan A. Safety and efficacy of N-acetylcysteine in children with non-acetaminophen-induced acute liver failure. *Liver Transpl.* 2008;14:25-30.
4. Lee WM, Hynan LS, Rossaro L, et al. Intravenous N-acetylcysteine improves transplant-free survival in early stage non-acetaminophen acute liver failure. *Gastroenterology.* 2009;137:856-864.
5. Ostapowicz G, Fontana RJ, Schiødt FV, et al. Results of a prospective study of acute liver failure at 17 tertiary care centers in the United States. *Ann Intern Med.* 2002;137:945-954.
6. Sklar GE, Subramaniam M. Acetylcysteine treatment for non-acetaminophen-induced acute liver failure. *Ann Pharmacother.* 2004;38:498-500.
7. Ben-Ari Z, Vaknin H, Tur-Kaspa R. N-acetylcysteine in acute hepatic failure (non-paracetamol-induced). *Hepatogastroenterology.* 2000;47:786-789.
8. Mumtaz K, Azam Z, Hamid S, et al. Role of N-acetylcysteine in adults with non-acetaminophen-induced acute liver failure in a center without the facility of liver transplantation. *Hepatol Int.* 2009;3:563-570.
9. Walsh TS, Hopton P, Philips BJ, Mackenzie SJ, Lee A. The effect of N-acetylcysteine on oxygen transport and uptake in patients with fulminant hepatic failure. *Hepatology.* 1998;27:1332-1340.

Should Living Donor Transplantation Be Considered in Adult Acute Liver Failure?

AnnMarie Liapakis, MD; Julia Wattacheril, MD, MPH; and Robert S. Brown Jr, MD, MPH

Acute liver failure (ALF) is a syndrome of severe acute liver injury with impaired synthetic function and encephalopathy in a person who previously had a normal liver or had well-compensated liver disease. The etiologies include drugs and toxins (particularly acetaminophen), viral, autoimmune, and other conditions. Other than a few direct antidotes (eg, N-acetylcysteine for acetaminophen overdose) there are no medical therapies for ALF and the mortality from this illness is high. It is estimated that there are approximately 2000 cases of ALF in the United States annually. Although relatively uncommon, ALF is associated with a poor prognosis. Medical supportive care alone leads to a spontaneous recovery in less than half of patients. Though patients have the highest status for transplantation, United Network of Organ Sharing (UNOS) Status 1, and are offered broader sharing than patients with chronic liver disease, mortality while waiting is high due to the rapid evolution of the disease and the development of cerebral edema. The rapid progression of ALF and shortage of available organs limits its effectiveness. Utilization of living donor liver transplantation (LDLT) could potentially overcome this organ shortage but is fraught with challenges. The need for a rapid donor decision, concern for potential coercion, and incomplete medical evaluations that might underestimate donor risk has led to reluctance to utilize LDLT for ALF. In fact some, including the guidelines of the New York State Health Department, consider ALF as a contraindication for LDLT. Additionally, the need for experienced centers may limit the applicability of this technique to many patients with ALF. These concerns have to be weighed against the high mortality of ALF patients on the waiting list, which likely could be decreased by a rapid transplant with a living donor. The current available data supports that the success rate and donor complication rate of LDLT is equivocal to that of DDLT for ALF and LDLT for chronic liver disease, respectively. This review highlights the data and the controversy in the use of LDLT for ALF in the United States.

Jensen D.
Controversies in Hepatology: The Experts Analyze Both Sides (pp 19-30)
© 2011 SLACK Incorporated

POINT

Acute Liver Failure Is a Catastrophic Illness With Significant Mortality and Limited Treatment Options

by AnnMarie Liapakis, MD

ALF refers to the rapid development of severe acute liver injury with impaired synthetic function and encephalopathy in a person who previously had a normal liver or had well-compensated liver disease. The duration between the onset of jaundice and development of encephalopathy further define it as hyperacute, 7 days; acute, 8 to 28 days; or subacute, >28 days to 12 weeks.[1] It is estimated that there are approximately 2000 cases of ALF in the United States annually.[2] Although relatively uncommon, ALF is associated with a poor prognosis. Medical supportive care alone leads to a spontaneous recovery in less than half of patients with ALF, with a transplant-free survival rate quoted at 43% in the largest prospective analysis in the United States, to date.[3] The rates differ by etiology with better survival for acetaminophen-related liver failure at 68% and lower for other drug reactions and liver failure of indeterminate cause at 25% and 17%, respectively, as shown in Figure 3-1.[3] Although there has been increasing interest in and study of artificial hepatic support systems, none of these devices is approved or has shown convincing efficacy in ALF. Therefore, liver transplantation remains the only current effective directed therapy.[4] Unfortunately, the rapid progression of ALF and shortage of available organs limit its effectiveness, despite giving patients with ALF the highest priority for transplant. Patients in the United States are listed as UNOS Status 1, which allows broader sharing of organs and priority above all patients with chronic liver failure. Despite this, 30 patients died between January 1998 and May 2001 across 17 tertiary care liver centers in the United States while awaiting a graft as a Status 1 on the UNOS list.[3] Utilization of living donor donation could overcome this organ shortage and decrease the mortality of this devastating condition. The need for a rapid donor decision—and concern that arose after a widely publicized donor death—has led to reluctance to utilize LDLT for ALF. In fact, some entities (including the New York State Health Department, according to their guidelines) consider acute liver failure as a contraindication for LDLT.[5,6] Though concern for coercion of the donor is real, the current evidence base supports that the success rate of LDLT is equivocal to that of deceased donor liver transplant (DDLT) for ALF, the donor complication rate in ALF is comparable to that of the complication rate in chronic liver disease, and LDLT offers an advantage over DDLT and opportunity to decrease the mortality of ALF. Therefore, LDLT should be reconsidered as an accepted therapy for ALF in the United States.

The Success Rate of Living Donor Liver Transplant Is Equivocal to That of Deceased Donor Liver Transplant for Acute Liver Failure

Substantial clinical experience, mostly outside the United States, utilizing LDLT for adult ALF has repeatedly demonstrated efficacy. A summary of this success is provided in Table 3-1.[7-9] One of the largest experiences reported is from Kyushu University Hospital in Japan where 42 LDLTs were performed (3 pediatric, 39 adult) for ALF between October

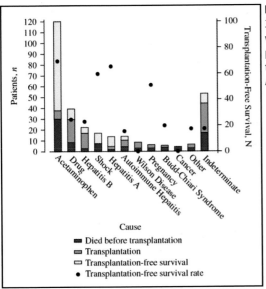

Figure 3-1. Presumed causes and outcomes in 308 patients with acute liver failure. (Reprinted with permission from Ostapowicz G. Results of a prospective study of acute liver failure at 17 tertiary care centers in the United States. *Ann Intern Med.* 2002;137:947-954.)

Table 3-1.

REPORTS OF LIVING DONOR LIVER TRANSPLANTATION FOR ACUTE LIVER FAILURE

AUTHOR	YEAR	CITY	TOTAL CASES	ADULT CASES	GRAFT L/R	1-YEAR SURVIVAL
Milwa	1999	Nagano	14	3	14/0	93% (13/14)
Lo	1999	Hong Kong	13	13	4/9	85% (11/13)
Uemoto	2000	Kyoto	34	15	26/8	59% (20/34)
Nishizaki	2002	Fukouka	15	15	15/0	80% (12/15)
Liu	2003	Hong Kong	16	16	0/16	88% (14/16)
Lubezky	2004	Tel Aviv	3	3	1/2	100% (3/3)
Wu	2004	Taipei	8	8	0/8	100% (8/8)
Lee	2007	Seoul	57	57	9/33*	82% (47/57)
Kilic	2007	Izmir	14	6	7/7	79% (11/14)
Ikegami	2008	Fukouka	42	39	31/8	78% (33/42)
Matsui	2008	Tokyo	36	32	16/18**	94% (34/36)
Campsen	2008	Various US	10	10	0/10	70% (7/10)

1996 and March 2007. The 1- and 10-year survival rates in this patient population, which included 12 hepatitis B patients, 1 hepatitis C patient, 2 autoimmune hepatitis patients, 3 Wilson's disease patients, and 24 unknown patients who were transplanted with a graft volume to standard liver volume ratio of greater than 35% (1 left lateral segment, 33 left lobe, 8 right lobe), were 80.0% and 68.2%, respectively, and 77.6% and 65.5%, respectively, for grafts.[9] Complication rates have been reported to be equivocal in LDLT when performed for ALF and for chronic liver disease in Japan, as illustrated in Table 3-2 in a report by Matsui.[8]

Table 3-2.			
COMPARISON OF COMPLICATIONS ENCOUNTERED IN ACUTE LIVER FAILURE AND NON-ACUTE LIVER FAILURE PATIENTS			
COMPLICATIONS	FULMINANT HEPATIC FAILURE (N=36)	NON-FULMINANT HEPATIC FAILURE (N=366)	P-VALUE
Acute cellular rejection	12 (33%)	116 (32%)	0.84
Hepatic arterial thrombosis	4 (11%)	17 (5%)	0.10
Portal venous thrombosis	2 (6%)	35 (10%)	0.43
Hepatic vein structure	1 (3%)	9 (2%)	0.91
Bile leakage	6 (17%)	58 (16%)	0.90
Biliary stricture	8 (22%)	73 (20%)	0.75
Total complication	23/36 (64%)	224/370 (61%)	0.75

*16 cases with dual graft noticed; **2 cases with lateral sector graft noticed.
(Reprinted with permission from Matsui Y. Living donor liver transplant for fulminant hepatic failure. *Hepatol Res.* 2008;38:987-996.)

Figure 3-2. Outcome of 14 patients with acute liver failure evaluated for LDLT. (Reprinted with permission from Campsen J, Blei AT, Emond JC, et al. Outcomes of living donor liver transplantation for acute liver failure: the adult-to-adult living donor liver transplantation cohort study. *Liver Transpl.* 2008;14(9):1273-1280.

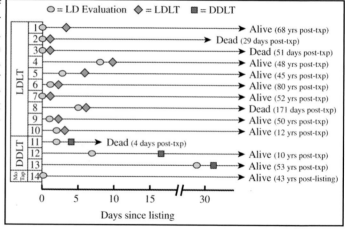

Since the first case of successful living-related liver transplantation in an adult with ALF in the United States documented by Kato in 1997, there has been a limited, but parallel, experience in Asia.[10] As part of the Adult to Adult Living Donor Liver Transplantation Cohort (A2ALL) study, outcomes of LDLT for ALF were reported from 9 US transplant centers. Fourteen patients (1% of the cohort) with ALF as the indication for transplant included 2 hepatitis A patients, 1 hepatitis B patient, 1 autoimmune hepatitis patient, 1 Wilson's disease patient, 1 acetaminophen toxicity patient, and 8 indeterminate cases who had a donor evaluated for potential LDLT. Of these, 10 patients received LDLT with a right hepatic lobe graft and 3 underwent DDLT (one clinically improved and was removed from the waiting list). As illustrated in Figure 3-2, the survival rates over a median of 5 years after LDLT (70%) and DDLT (67%) were equivalent.[9] When compared to survival rates of DDLT, this 70% survival rate of LDLT in ALF is similar to the 82% survival rate of DDLT in ALF reported by the Organ Procurement and Transplantation Network that same year. Farmer et al reviewed a 17-year experience with 204 patients who underwent liver transplant for ALF at Dumont-UCLA Transplant Center and reported 1- and 5-year survival rates of 73% and 67%, which is equivocal to that of the LDLTs in A2ALL. Five percent of this UCLA population included living donor of left lateral segments and ex vivo-reduced cadaveric grafts. On univariate analysis conducted to identify pre-transplant factors that would predict outcome, the authors concluded that donor graft type was not predictive of patient survival.[11] In addition to equivalent post-transplant survival, it would be expected that LDLT would improve overall survival by reducing the risk of death on the waiting list and allowing optimal timing of transplant after it was determined that spontaneous recovery was unlikely.

One concern about critically ill recipients receiving a partial graft is the development of "small-for-size syndrome," with portal hypertension, cholestasis, and liver failure post-LDLT. Importantly, unlike patients with chronic liver failure and high model for end-stage liver disease (MELD) score, none of the patients with ALF in A2ALL had small-for-size syndrome. The concern that ALF patients are too sick to tolerate a partial graft from a living donor was also refuted by Ikegami who reported a patient who successfully received only 25% of the estimated standard liver volume. The authors suggest that patients with ALF may actually tolerate smaller liver volumes as they have no pre-existing portal hypertension.[12,13]

The Donor Complication Rate of Living Donor Liver Transplant in Acute Liver Failure Is Comparable to That of Living Donor Liver Transplant in Chronic Liver Disease

It is established that donor evaluation in the setting of ALF can be completed within half of a day. Though care has to be taken to exclude coercion, this necessary expedited evaluation has not led to an increase in donor complications due to missed medical conditions.

In the A2ALL study, the rate of complications in donors in ALF (50%) was comparable to the rate of complications in donors for all indications (37.7%), and donor perioperative survival was 100%.[9] Of note was the fact that there were no severe psychological complications reported in the 10 donors in ALF as compared to 4% in the A2ALL study. Previously, severe psychological complications have been raised as a concern given limited donor evaluation time in ALF. Our experience is that the donors who volunteer in this scenario are usually closely related (parents, spouses, adult children, siblings) and thus coercion may be less of an issue than some more distantly related donor volunteers in chronic cases.

In the largest series of LDLT for ALF abroad, there was no increase in donor complication rate over that of LDLT for chronic liver disease. Lee, who reported a series of 57 cases at the Asan Medical Center in Korea, stated that "none of the donors suffered from major complications apartfrom one who developed an intrahepatic pseudoaneurysm after percutaneous needle biopsy" that was treated successfully.[14] Ikegami in Japan reported a donor complication rate of 35.7%, which is equivocal to that reported for all donors in the A2ALL study in the United States. Complications were for the most part mild, including bile duct stenosis or injury (3 cases), persistent hyperbilirubinemia (2 cases), peptic ulcer disease (2 cases), gastric stasis (3 cases), wound problems (3 cases), alopecia (1 case), and temporary ulnar palsy (1 case). This is likely an acceptable price to donors to be able to save the life of a loved one. There were no donor deaths.[12] Similarly, Matsui reported only 2 donor complications, including one bile leak and one case of delayed gastric emptying.[8]

The initial fear that a rapid evaluation would miss medical or surgical issues leading to an increased donor complication rate with right lobe liver donation has been refuted. Liu established right lobe live donor liver transplantation (the procedure that has been pursued in the

United States) as a treatment option for patients with ALF. He reported a low donor morbidity, including only 3 wound infections, 1 peroneal nerve palsy, and no donor deaths.[15]

Living Donor Liver Transplantation Offers an Advantage Over Deceased Donor Liver Transplantation

LDLT offers the benefit of being able to more appropriately time transplantation and avoid the death of listed patients while awaiting a graft. This benefit has been documented in both chronic liver disease and ALF. For ALF, Liu et al showed that compared with a group of patients without donor volunteers, those who had a donor evaluated for potential LDLT had a higher chance of receiving a transplant (19 of 34 versus 1 of 16) and survival (17 of 34 versus 1 of 16).[15] Similarly, the zero mortality of ALF patients on the waiting list in A2ALL was in sharp comparison to that of a 22% mortality reported by Ostapowicz with DDLT.[16]

LDLT obviates the need to potentially accept a marginally deceased donor whole liver graft, which is often accepted as extended criteria donors to overcome prohibitive wait times. This has resulted in a high rate of primary graft nonfunction (PNF) in some series (eg, 13.2% reported by Farmer).[11] Living donor grafts are uniformly good quality with low rates of PNF.[16] Having a living donor available also allows one to bypass an organ offer when there is still a chance of spontaneous recovery without the fear that no organs will be available if the disease progresses or cerebral edema develops, allowing optimal timing for transplant.

Summary

Substantial experience abroad and recent smaller, parallel domestic trials utilizing LDLT for adult ALF document excellent post-transplant survival and acceptable complication rates in consideration of the substantial organ shortage. LDLT should be considered in the setting of ALF in the United States and guidelines re-examined. Ultimately, refinement of LDLT application and technique in ALF can further optimize outcomes.

KEY POINTS

- There are limited treatment options in ALF.
- The success rate of LDLT in ALF is equal to non-ALF.
- Donor complication in ALF is equal to ESLD.
- LDLT allows optimal timing of transplant in ALF.
- LDLT obviates the need to accept marginal grafts.

COUNTERPOINT

Living Donor Liver Transplantation in Acute Liver Failure Represents Unethical Coercion With Suboptimal Outcomes When Adequate Alternatives Exist

by Julia Wattacheril, MD, MPH

ALF, or the rapid (less than 2 weeks) onset of encephalopathy following the clinical development of jaundice, is a medical urgency that carries a high mortality without intervention, namely liver transplantation. While we can agree that the need for better therapies exist in ALF, the case for living donor transplantation in this circumstance is fraught with obstacles. The most harrowing of which is an ethical issue that is applicable to living donation liver transplantation (LDLT) under any circumstance; the potential violation of the principle of nonmaleficence, the first dictum of medicine: that is, to do no harm. The donor is exposed to risk from a surgical procedure of no medical necessity without obtaining any physical benefit. The need for rapid evaluation makes matters worse, with the donor having inadequate time to weigh the risks of the decision. Furthermore, LDLT under any circumstance should also be considered unethical when performed at centers with suboptimal facilities or expertise, which would further limit applicability of LDLT for ALF. While a survival benefit has been demonstrated in individuals on the waiting list who pursue LDLT, this has only been shown in a convincing manner for those with chronic liver failure.[21] Pursuant to the ethical hurdles come psychological, cultural, medical, logistical, and financial problems that render LDLT for ALF a risky alternative to deceased donor liver transplantation (DDLT).

Ethical Issues for the Donor

Freedom from coercion remains an important consideration in the process of donor assessment and one reason our center assigns each potential living donor an independent donor assessment team.[22] The evaluation climate and pace varies considerably between chronic liver disease and ALF transplant candidates. Most transplant evaluations take place over a period of weeks to months, whereas the rapid evaluation required in ALF takes hours to days. Coercion is defined by the 2010 Random House Dictionary[23] as "domination or controlling [an individual] especially by exploiting fear, anxiety, etc." As accepted donors are typically biological relatives or close friends of the recipient, donation during the emotionally charged and dramatic presentation of ALF carries significant risk of unintended coercion. The most common donor candidates in the Adult to Adult Living Donor Liver Transplantation (A2ALL) cohort were offspring of the recipient (34% all potential donors, 31% of accepted donors).[1,24] The psychological toll of a relative facing imminent death may be sufficient-enough emotional context for coercion to be felt on the part of the donor. The role of the psychosocial team in determining suitability is limited by the expediency of the evaluation. It is estimated that at least 15% of potential donors choose not to pursue further evaluation after just one initial meeting.[25,26] Significant ongoing donor dropout occurs throughout the evaluation process. A truncated process may therefore capture medically appropriate donors who might otherwise, given time for careful consideration and ongoing informed consent, reconsider their decision. While the psychosocial assessment of the recipient is often incomplete given the paucity of clear information in many cases of ALF, the donor assessment cannot afford that risk. The donor must be able to exercise his or her autonomy to decline evaluation or proceeding with donation without guilt. This has led to guidelines including a 2-week "cooling off" period after donor acceptance to allow the donor to reconsider, which would be unfeasible in cases of ALF. Additionally, expanding the indications of living donation to include cases of ALF, while increasing the donor pool, may place additional burdens on an already distressed recipient psychosocial support system.

Psychological Issues

Hayashi et al[27] found that the psychological status of donors was not related to the characteristics of the donor or recipient medical conditions but was relevant to decision-making motivation and process of donation; similarly, factors that contributed to donors' quality of life (QOL) were mostly state-trait anxiety and environmental QOL. State-trait anxiety relates to situational anxiety surrounding an event (ie, ALF in a loved one) as opposed to anxiety traits (chronic anxiety).[27] These psychological factors are not insignificant or easily ameliorated. In fact, in review of 392 A2ALL donors, 16 (4.1%) had one or multiple psychiatric complications post donation, including 3 severe psychiatric complications (suicide, accidental drug overdose, and suicide attempt). The psychosocial screening process must not be cursory or rushed given these grave implications.[28]

Outcomes Vary Based on Center Experience

While the data from Asian countries is upheld as sufficient justification for limited morbidity and mortality in donors following donation, the numerator is not the only concern. The overall experience with living donation (for all indications, not just ALF) in Asian countries is much higher than in Western countries, especially in the United States. Increased experience has been shown to decrease complication rates, but many centers in the United States would have inadequate experience to perform LDLT for ALF and there is no opportunity for potential recipients to travel to experienced centers in most cases of ALF. Even in experienced centers, the morbidity associated with right graft harvesting is not negligible. In 2006, Middleton et al[29] systematically reviewed the morbidity and mortality of living donation liver transplantation worldwide. Overall reported donor mortality in 117 studies was 12 to 13 cases in about 6000 procedures (0.2%). Mortality for right lobe donors to adult recipients was estimated to be 2 to 8 out of 3800 (0.23% to 0.5%). The donor morbidity rate ranged from 0% to 100% with a median of 16% in 131 studies. Biliary complications and infections were the most commonly reported donor morbidities.[2,29] These morbidities must be seen in the background of 0% donor morbidity with the alternative of no LDLT and only using deceased donors.

Despite center experience, certain technical complications occur. In Japan where deceased donation is rare for cultural reasons and living donation is often the only option for transplantation, Hashikura et al[30] reviewed the complication rates of 38 centers (3565 living donors). Preoperative problems were reported in 2 donors, intraoperative problems in 27 donors, and postoperative complications in 270 donors. In total, 299 donors (8.4%) suffered complications related to liver donation. Postoperative complications included biliary complications in 3.0%, reoperation in 1.3%, severe after-effects in 2 donors (0.06%), and death apparently related to donor surgery in 1 donor (0.03%). The incidence of postoperative complications in left- and right-lobe donors was 8.7% and 9.4%, respectively.[30] While risks can be minimized, they cannot be eliminated. Justifying this risk in the setting of ALF then becomes incumbent on equivalent, or even superior, outcomes for the recipient.

Graft and Recipient Outcomes in Fulminant Hepatic Failure

Adult to adult living donation for fulminant hepatic failure (FHF) is not common in the West. FHF is defined as acute hepatocellular necrosis complicated by the development of hepatic encephalopathy within 8 weeks of the onset of jaundice. In 2000, Uemoto et al[18] evaluated 38 patients (both adult and pediatric) who presented with and underwent living donor transplantation. Thirty-six donor operations, including 2 retransplantations for ductopenic rejection and refractory acute rejection, were performed for 34 recipients (19 patients less than 18 years old and 15 adults). The outcomes were significantly worse than LDLT for other indications. Overall patient survival at 1, 2, and 3 years after LDLT was 59%. Graft survival at the same time points was 56%.[18] Justifying donor risk for these outcomes in a center with high rates of LDLT seems difficult. While Campsen may have shown similar 5-year survival between LDLT and DDLT in those patients undergoing transplantation for ALF,[11] it should be noted that these patients comprised only 1% of the cohort (10 undergoing LDLT and 3 DDLT); it is dangerous to draw significant conclusions from such small samples.

Summary

LDLT offers many individuals shorter wait times and contributes to improved survival in patients with chronic liver disease. However, though its use in acute liver failure may indeed decrease waiting times in a medically urgent setting, the risk/benefit ratio is much narrower, even in experienced centers. Given the rarity of the disease, few cases will even be at centers with adequate experience, thus the potential benefit is smaller. Excluding donor coercion is difficult if not impossible, and the potential for serious donor medical and psychological harm exists without adequate time for the donor to make an informed and autonomous decision. Finally, in the United States, expedited access to transplant with UNOS Status 1 allows prompt transplant. Even broader sharing of deceased donor grafts for ALF would likely reduce waiting list mortality far more than the use of LDLT in this setting. Thus, LDLT should likely be reserved for non-acute settings and should not be utilized in acute liver failure.

KEY POINTS

- The catastrophe of ALF and rapid donor evaluation leads to donor coercion.
- The psychosocial stress donors face have long-term sequelae.
- Outcomes in LDLT for ALF vary with a center's experience.
- Outcomes are worse in ALF than LDLT for other indications.

EXPERT OPINION

Living Donor Liver Transplantation for Acute Liver Failure: Proceed, But With Extreme Caution

by Robert S. Brown Jr, MD, MPH

A central tenet in medicine is *primum non nocere*, first do no harm. On the surface, LDLT contradicts this principle, because a healthy individual undergoes a major operation for no direct, physical benefit. However, this is only if one uses a narrow definition of benefit. Since LDLT has now been shown to provide survival benefit to the recipient, donation will also benefit the donor if they are emotionally linked to recipient outcome.

The first adult-to-adult LDLT was performed in Hong Kong in 1993. Five years later, the first LDLT was performed in the United States, and, today, there are over 90 centers that have performed at least one LDLT across the country, though most are done in a smaller number of larger-volume centers. In other parts of the world where deceased donor transplant is unavailable or severely limited, particularly Asia, the majority of transplants and transplant centers use LDLT. In the US, the volume has stabilized at ~250/cases per year, about half of the peak in 2001, and less than 5% of total transplants. Worldwide, the number of LDLTs performed and centers performing it continues to grow, highlighting that demand for the procedure has not changed. However, very few of these cases have been done for ALF, particularly in the United States.

At the current time, most experts concur that recipients considered for LDLT should fulfill the same criteria established for deceased donor liver transplantation. Some transplant physicians and surgeons believe that LDLT should be extended to patients not felt to be candidates for deceased donor grafts (eg, metastatic tumors, acute alcoholic hepatitis, or in urgent situations such as patients with high MELD score and acute liver failure). This, unfortunately, raises several ethical issues. The principle of autonomy should allow donors and recipients to make an independent decision even if the risk is prohibitive or a deceased donor transplant is felt contraindicated. Especially since in many of these situations the outcome for the recipient is still better than it would be without a transplant. And patients with acute liver failure are clearly candidates for a deceased donor graft in many situations.

The main ethical dilemma is assessing the level of acceptable risk of mortality to the donor and determining whether this is an absolute measure or one that is relative to the expected recipient outcome and the donor preferences. The risk of donor mortality is higher with LDLT than kidney donation. But this is a relative risk. The absolute risk is small and substantially less than the ~20% risk of mortality for all candidates on the waiting list. The waiting list mortality is substantially higher in many regions for patients with acute liver failure who need to receive a deceased donor graft within 1 to 4 days. The principle of autonomy places the perspective of the donor as the most important. The donor must be informed of the risks associated with the procedure. Coercion of the donor needs to be excluded during an independent, confidential evaluation. This can be difficult to accomplish in LDLT for ALF. Excluding coercion and ensuring an informed decision in a greatly compressed time frame is difficult. Additionally, a rapid donor evaluation may increase the likelihood of medical conditions being missed and thus underestimate the actual risk faced by the donor. However, the limited data available has not demonstrated higher donor complication rates for LDLT cases in urgent conditions.

Studies from the time of evaluation have all demonstrated substantial benefits of pursuing LDLT on waiting time mortality.[31-33] Patients are interested in their overall survival, not only if they survive to transplant. It appears that except for patients with high MELD scores, LDLT offers equivalent results to DDLT from the time of transplant at experienced centers, despite an initial belief that for any given severity of illness a whole organ should result in superior outcomes compared to a partial organ. This has not been as clearly established for ALF, but based on the available data, excellent results can be achieved with LDLT for ALF—perhaps comparable to DDLT—when done early in appropriate candidates. And the waiting list mortality for patients with ALF is higher than for most MELD scores even when listed as UNOS Status 1. Thus the benefit in terms of decreasing waiting list mortality may exceed that for patients with chronic liver failure. The longer the mean Status 1 or urgent waiting time for a deceased donor graft, the greater the potential benefit. Additionally, availability of LDLT allows clinicians to wait until recovery from ALF is not possible but before contraindications to OLT develop (eg, increased ICP). For DDLT, cases may be done too early due to fear that another organ may not be offered in time, or too late after cerebral edema or increased intracranial pressure has already developed. LDLT offer the opportunity to potentially optimize timing of transplant for ALF and potentially improve outcome for patients.

However, care has to be taken with the donor evaluation to ensure informed consent and lack of coercion. It also needs to be done promptly to avoid pressure to perform futile transplants when a patient has waited several days with progressive deterioration and no deceased donors are available. Likely the use of LDLT for ALF in the United States should be limited to donors who are closely emotionally linked (spouses, parents, first degree relatives) who volunteer immediately upon admission. Use of closely related individuals makes it less likely that there is coercion and increases the benefit to the donor. Patients should be appropriate candidates for DDLT and be listed as UNOS Status 1. At the current time, I would not offer LDLT to patients with contraindications to DDLT, as the degree of potential coercion is too great. Evaluation should be rapid (~48 hours) and include a careful psychosocial evaluation. Potential donors should understand the risks and that alternate therapies exist (ie, deceased donor transplant as UNOS Status 1). The transplant should be done after 72 to 96 hours when it is clear that there are no acceptable deceased donors readily available and that spontaneous liver recovery will not occur. Data should be collected on donor and recipient outcome including long-term donor satisfaction with their decision and QOL. If done correctly, I believe LDLT for ALF can be performed in select cases in an ethical way that is potentially life-saving as an adjunct to DDLT. Adult living donor liver transplantation offers improved access to a life-saving transplant for patients with end stage liver disease in areas where waiting time mortality is high and availability of deceased donor organs falls short of the need of the population. This principle is clearly met for chronic liver failure, and for many cases, is likely met for ALF.

References

1. Riordan SM. Fulminant hepatic failure. In: Schiff ER, ed. *Schiff's Diseases of the Liver*. 10th ed. Philadelphia, PA: Lippincott Williams & Wilkins; 2007:601-636.
2. Lee WM. Acute liver failure. *N Engl J Med*. 1993;329:1862-1872.
3. Ostapowicz G. Results of a prospective study of acute liver failure at 17 tertiary care centers in the United States. *Ann Intern Med*. 2002;137:947-954.
4. Hoofnagle JH. Fulminant hepatic failure: summary of a workshop. *Hepatology*. 1995;21:240-252.
5. Department of Health Press Release: www.health.state.ny.us/press/releases/2002/mtsinai.htm
6. Novello AC. New York State Committee on Quality Improvement in Living Liver Donation. Troy, NY: New York State Health Department; 2002.

7.   Akamatsu N. Acute liver failure and living donor liver transplantation. *Hepatol Res.* 2008;38(suppl): S60-S71.
8.   Matsui Y. Living donor liver transplant for fulminant hepatic failure. *Hepatol Res.* 2008;38:987-996.
9.   Campsen J, Blei AT, Emond JC, et al. Outcomes of living donor liver transplantation for acute liver failure: the adult-to-adult living donor liver transplantation cohort study. *Liver Transpl.* 2008;14(9):1273-1280.
10.   Kato T. Successful living related liver transplantation in an adult with fulminant hepatic failure. *Transplantation.* 1997;64:415-417.
11.   Farmer DG. Liver transplantation for fulminant hepatic failure: experience with more than 200 patients over a 17-yr period. *Ann Surg.* 2003;237:666-676.
12.   Ikegami T. Living donor liver transplantation for acute liver failure: a 10-year experience in a single center. *J Am Coll Surg.* 2008;206:411-418.
13.   Yonemura Y. Validity of preoperative volumetric analysis of congestion volume in living donor LT using three-dimensional computed tomography. *Liver Transplantation.* 2005;11:1556-1162.
14.   Lee SG. I prefer living donor liver transplantation. *J Hepatol.* 2007;46:553-582.
15.   Liu CL. Right-lobe live donor liver transplantation improves survival of patients with acute liver failure. *Br J Surg.* 2002;89:317-322.
16.   Chung-Mau L. Liver transplantation for acute liver failure: not too early but never too late. *Liver Transplantation.* 2008;14:1243-1244.
17.   Miwa S. Living-related liver transplantation for patients with fulminant and subfulminant hepatic failure. *Hepatology.* 1999;30:1521-1526.
18.   Uemoto S, Inomata Y, Sakurai T, et al. Living donor liver transplantation for fulminant hepatic failure. *Transplantation.* 2000;70(1):152-157.
19.   Lubezky N. Initial experience with urgent adult-to-adult living donor liver transplantation in fulminant hepatic failure. *Isr Med Assoc J.* 2004;6:467-470.
20.   Wu YM. Liver transplantation for acute hepatic failure. *Transplant Proc.* 2004;36:2226-2227.
21.   Berg CL, et al. Improvement in survival associated with adult-to-adult living donor liver transplantation. *Gastroenterol.* 2007;133(6):1806-1813.
22.   Brown RS Jr. Live donors in liver transplantation. *Gastroenterology.* 2008;134(6):1802-1813.
23.   coercion. Dictionary.com Unabridged. Random House, Inc. http://dictionary.reference.com/browse/coercion (accessed: April 03, 2011).
24.   Trotter JF, Wisniewski KA, Terrault NA, et al. Outcomes of donor evaluation in adult-to-adult living donor liver transplantation. *Hepatology.* 2007;46(5):1476-1484.
25.   Pomfret EA, Pomposelli JJ, Lewis WD, et al. Live donor adult liver transplantation using right lobe grafts: donor evaluation and surgical outcome. *Arch Surg.* 2001;136(4):425-433.
26.   Pomfret EA, Pomposelli JJ, Jenkins RL. Live donor liver transplantation. *J Hepatol.* 2001;34(4):613-624.
27.   Hayashi A, Noma S, Uehara M, et al. Relevant factors to psychological status of donors before living-related liver transplantation. *Transplantation.* 2007;84(10):1255-1261.
28.   Trotter JF, Hill-Callahan MM, Gillespie BW, et al. Severe psychiatric problems in right hepatic lobe donors for living donor liver transplantation. *Transplantation.* 2007;83(11):1506-1508.
29.   Middleton PF, Duffield M, Lynch SV, et al. Living donor liver transplantation, adult donor outcomes: a systematic review. *Liver Transpl.* 2006;12(1):24-30.
30.   Hashikura Y, Ichida T, Umeshita K, et al. Donor complications associated with living donor liver transplantation in Japan. *Transplantation.* 2009;88(1):110-114.
31.   Russo MW, LaPointe-Rudow D, Kinkhabwala M, Emond J, Brown RS, Jr. Impact of adult living donor liver transplantation on waiting time survival in candidates listed for liver transplantation. *Am J Transplant.* 2004;4(3):427-431.
32.   Berg CL, Gillespie BW, Merion RM, et al. Improvement in survival associated with adult-to-adult living donor liver transplantation. *Gastroenterology.* 2007;133(6):1806-1813.
33.   Liu CL, Lam B, Lo CM, Fan ST. Impact of right-lobe live donor liver transplantation on patients waiting for liver transplantation. *Liver Transpl.* 2003;9(8):863-869.

SECTION II
CHRONIC HEPATITIS B AND C

DO ALL PATIENTS WITH CHRONIC HEPATITIS B WHO ARE TREATMENT CANDIDATES NEED AN ASSESSMENT OF FIBROSIS?

Hector Nazario, MD; Carmen Landaverde, MD; and Robert Perrillo, MD

Liver biopsy is a time-honored tool in staging chronic viral hepatitis and has long been utilized by specialists to convey prognosis and assist in determining whether to treat chronic viral hepatitis. The last decade, however, has witnessed the development of multiple noninvasive means of determining liver fibrosis. In addition, more easily acceptable oral agents have become available that appear safe for long-term use. Published treatment guidelines from the major liver societies emphasize predefined biochemical and serum hepatitis B virus (HBV) DNA thresholds and are not very specific about the level of injury needed for treatment. It is not surprising, then, that the need for liver biopsy has recently become more controversial.

In this chapter, Drs. Hector Nazario and Carmen Landaverde discuss the advantages and limitations of liver biopsy with particular emphasis on how this affects treatment decisions and whether this is a prerequisite to making the best decision.

POINT

A Liver Biopsy Is Generally Necessary When Making a Decision to Treat Patients With Chronic Hepatitis B

by Hector Nazario, MD

Determining the stage of fibrosis has important clinical implications because it is the most relevant histological prognostic factor in chronic hepatitis B (HBV). Patients with stage III or

Jensen D.
Controversies in Hepatology: The Experts Analyze Both Sides (pp 33-42)
© 2011 SLACK Incorporated

stage IV disease are at greater risk of long-term complications such as liver failure and hepatocellular carcinoma (HCC) and, correspondingly, they have a greater requirement for antiviral therapy. By contrast, individuals with stage 0 to I fibrosis are less apt to need treatment, particularly if longstanding infection is suspected. While several blood tests that measure hyaluronic acid or other elements of collagen matrix are currently available to measure the degree of fibrosis, these tests suffer from lower accuracy in patients with intermediate levels of fibrosis.[1,2] Also, as these tests are not disease specific, they have limited value in situations where more than one source of liver injury is present (ie, fatty liver and viral hepatitis).

There has been growing interest in transient elastography, or FibroScan (EchoSens, Paris, France). Several studies have shown good correlation with the results of liver biopsy in chronic HBV and a variety of other liver disorders.[3-5] However, the diagnostic accuracy of transient elastography is still undergoing investigation and needs further validation before it can be considered a reliable alternative for determining the extent of fibrosis. Moreover, signal intensity is affected by necroinflammation, congestion, cholestasis, and possibly even steatosis.[6,7] In one large study, liver stiffness measurements were judged to be uninterpretable in nearly 1 in 5 cases, principally due to obesity.[8] Thus, liver biopsy remains the gold standard for evaluating the degree of fibrosis and remains necessary in most patients who are being considered for treatment.

Clinical Utility of Liver Biopsy Goes Beyond Staging

There are several advantages to liver biopsy other than obtaining information on the stage of fibrosis. A baseline appraisal of liver histology can provide valuable information on coexisting liver diseases that may be present.[9] This can alter the therapeutic approach.

Although newer nucleoside analogues have greater antiviral potency, the rate of treatment response is still suboptimal and long-term treatment is often necessary.[10] The extended duration of treatment has implications for safety as well as cost of care and underscores the need for careful selection of patients who have more than minimal liver disease.

Neither alanine aminotransferase (ALT) level nor degree of viral replication correlates with the extent of fibrosis, and both parameters can fluctuate widely in HBeAg-negative chronic hepatitis B.[9,11] As a result, observation at 3-month intervals is recommended for HBeAg-negative patients during the first year to distinguish them from inactive HBsAg carriers.[12] Patients with HBeAg-negative chronic HBV generally have longstanding infection, however, and there is a greater risk for cirrhosis. As liver biopsy depicts the effects of accumulative organ damage, it can expedite an earlier treatment decision in patients with fluctuating disease.

Staging Patients With Viral Coinfections

Patients who are coinfected with hepatitis C virus, human immunodeficiency virus (HIV), or hepatitis D virus have been shown to have an accelerated course of disease and are at greater risk for cirrhosis.[13-15] Thus, liver biopsy is more apt to reveal advanced fibrosis in these patients. HIV-infected patients have greatly lengthened survival with current highly active antiretroviral therapy (HAART) regimens, thus making liver disease a more common cause of death.[16] The use of nucleotide-containing regimens with activity against HBV have been shown to effectively control viral replication in these patients.[16] However, treatment compliance has been shown to be suboptimal in HIV-infected patients and demonstration of severe fibrosis could encourage better compliance, thereby minimizing the chance for drug-resistant HBV mutants.[17]

Limitations of Current Alanine Aminotransferase Thresholds to Assess Liver Injury

Current international management guidelines for HBV recommend treatment selection that is based on the degree of ALT elevation (>2 x ULN) and level of viremia (>20,000 IU/mL for HBeAg-positive patients and >2,000 IU for HBeAg-negative patients).[12,18-20] Several independent studies, however, have shown that as many as 30% of HBsAg carriers who meet the HBV DNA criteria but not the recommended ALT threshold can have greater than or equal to grade II and greater than or equal to stage II injury.[21-25] These patients often tend to be middle aged, HBeAg-negative, and of Asian ethnicity, suggesting that HBV infection was acquired in early life. Only liver biopsy can establish the true extent of liver injury in these patients.

It has also been shown that the finding of normal ALT can be misleading because standard laboratory reference ranges reflect mean values found in obese, diabetic, or ethanol-consuming individuals without a known history of liver disease. Of these, perhaps the most important confounding patient-related variable is body mass index.[26,27] Asian HBsAg carriers tend to be considerably leaner than White and African American carriers. Accordingly, their true normal ALT levels are generally lower. To adjust for these factors, more stringent limits for the upper limit of normal (19 IU for females, 30 IU for males) have been advocated by several health authorities and are recommended in the American Association for the Study of Liver Diseases (AASLD) Practice Guidelines.[12,28,29]

Summary

Liver biopsy remains the best tool to determine the prognosis of an individual with HBV and the need for treatment. Oral antiviral therapy for HBV is expensive and needs to be given for extended periods, perhaps indefinitely. Thus, selection of patients who are likely to benefit most will continue to be important and liver biopsy remains an important tool in this process. ALT criteria have been established for treatment, but some patients with moderately severe liver disease are not being identified using the recommended ranges of abnormality. Part of this discrepancy reflects inaccurate assessment of the upper limit of normal, and this can be rectified by the use of new limits that reflect values in patients with healthy livers. Unfortunately, these have not been adopted by most commercial laboratories. Until these new norms are adopted, a broader rather than a more restrictive use of liver biopsy will help identify additional patients who may potentially benefit from treatment.

KEY POINTS

- Liver biopsy is the gold standard for evaluation of fibrosis stage.
- Liver biopsy can establish contribution of liver injury from coexisting liver disease.
- Liver biopsy determines cumulative damage in patients with longstanding infection.
- Liver biopsy identifies "moderate hepatitis" in those who do not meet ALT criteria.
- Liver biopsy encourages treatment adherence in those with significant injury.

A Liver Biopsy Is Not Essential When Making a Decision to Treat Patients With Chronic Hepatitis B

by Carmen Landaverde, MD

A liver biopsy can be a valuable tool in the clinical management of chronic hepatitis B (HBV). It provides information on the extent of inflammation and fibrosis and may enable early identification of unsuspected cirrhosis. The latter, in turn, may define a need for earlier surveillance for HCC. As pointed out by Dr. Nazario, biopsy occasionally may be helpful in excluding other common causes of liver disease such as fatty liver. However, I contend that liver biopsy is not an absolute prerequisite when making a decision to provide antiviral therapy.

Current Management Guidelines Do Not Recommend All Treatment Candidates to Have a Liver Biopsy Prior to Initiating Therapy

The recommendations made in the management guidelines for HBV that have been sponsored by the major liver societies, both in the United States and abroad, support this position.[12,18,19] For example, the AASLD Practice Guidelines indicate that a liver biopsy is optional and most useful in persons who do not meet clear cut ALT guidelines discussed above.[12] The guidelines provide the example of a patient over the age of 40 (presumably one exposed early in life) who has appropriate levels of serum HBV DNA but minimally elevated or even normal ALT values. Rendering final judgment on the issue of biopsy is left to the clinician. While the Clinical Practice Guidelines of the European Association for the Study of the Liver (EASL) recommend liver biopsy as a means of assisting the decision to use antiviral therapy, the panel of experts is careful to point out that it is usually not required in patients with clinical evidence of cirrhosis nor in those in whom treatment is indicated for other reasons.[18] Also, a treatment algorithm by an expert panel suggested that a liver biopsy is not mandatory in patients with intermittent or persistent ALT elevation and HBV DNA levels equal to or greater than 10^4 or 10^5 copies/mL, depending on HBeAg status.[20] Instead, the authors emphasize that a liver biopsy might be especially useful in HBsAg carriers with normal ALT levels who are over the age of 35. Thus, while these recommendations vary somewhat, there is relatively uniform agreement that patients who meet ALT and HBV DNA criteria or have obvious features of moderate to severe hepatitis or cirrhosis should be treated and do not require liver biopsy.

Patients at High Risk of Hepatocellular Carcinoma or Disease Progression May Be Treated Without Prior Assessment of Fibrosis

The decision to treat is based on a number of factors and, in some patients, a positive decision may hinge on the assessed risk for future complications–if there is a family history of hepatocellular carcinoma (HCC) or when a progressive decline in platelet count and splenomegaly signals the emergence of portal hypertension. It is well established that individuals with chronic HBV who have a positive family history of HCC have a significantly higher risk of developing HCC.[30,31] A recent case-control study found patients with a positive family history of HCC to have a 4-fold increased risk.[31]

There are also subsets of patients in which the importance of a liver biopsy is not specifically addressed in current treatment guidelines. An example of this can be found in patients with HBV who are coinfected with hepatitis C virus, hepatitis delta virus, or human immunodeficiency virus (HIV). These patients have a much greater risk not only for progressive liver disease and liver failure but also liver cancer.[32] Therefore, if criteria are met for ALT and HBV DNA, liver biopsy may not add much to the clinical decision. Another group where biopsy may provide limited additional information needed to render a treatment decision is found in individuals with multiple risk factors for HCC. In addition to coinfection with other viruses and a positive family history, this includes male gender, older age, high HBV DNA level, history of reversion from anti-HBe to HBeAg, core promoter mutation, and HBV genotype C.[33-36]

Procedure-Related Factors Can Influence the Decision to Perform a Liver Biopsy

While liver biopsy is generally safe, it is an invasive procedure with small but definite associated risks. For example, an evaluation of 2740 liver biopsies in the Hepatitis C Antiviral Long-Term Treatment Against Cirrhosis (HALT-C) trial revealed that serious adverse events occurred in 1.1% of all liver biopsies with no associated deaths.[37] The most common serious event was bleeding with a frequency of 0.6%, and patients with a platelet count of 60,000/mm^3 or less had the highest risk of bleeding. Pain after a percutaneous liver biopsy is frequently reported, occurring in approximately 85% of patients.[38] One must also consider that certain patients may have contraindications to liver biopsy due to anatomical factors, significant coagulopathy, coexisting infection in the hepatic bed, or extrahepatic biliary obstruction.[38] To justify the liver biopsy-associated risks, it is imperative that the sample obtained is adequate for interpretation. A specimen length of at least 20 mm in length (obtained with a 16-gauge needle) is considered a reliable size for grading and staging in chronic viral hepatitis.[39-41] However, even when performed by experienced hepatologists, one study reported that only 23% of the biopsy specimens were at least 20 mm in length.[40] This increases the chance for inaccurate assessment of the degree of fibrosis.[41] Therefore, one has to be mindful of the inherent procedure risks, patient factors that put a particular individual at increased risk of complications, and the likelihood of obtaining an adequate sample size for accurate interpretation before recommending a liver biopsy.

Antiviral Therapy Is Effective and Associated With Histologic Benefit

The benefits of antiviral therapy in the treatment of chronic HBV are well established. The registration trials for all of the currently available antiviral agents have shown improved histologic outcomes in responders.[9] Newer oral antiviral agents have greater potency and nominal rates of drug resistance. Thus, when compared to lamivudine and adefovir, current nucleoside analog therapy should lead to even better outcomes in terms of achieving a decline in the rate of hepatic decompensation, need for liver transplantation, evolution to HCC, and improved survival.[42] It can be argued, therefore, that liver biopsy is less relevant for those in whom there are obvious clinical or laboratory features that prompt initiation of treatment but more relevant as a tool to monitor disease progression in patients who cannot be successfully treated.

Summary

The decision to perform a liver biopsy before initiation of antiviral therapy is best done when it is individualized. It is clear that not all patients require a liver biopsy in order for a sound clinical decision to be made. While traditionally considered important for prognostic determination, new therapies have become more effective and histologic improvement can be anticipated whenever a virologic response is either maintained during treatment or is found to be durable after treatment has been discontinued.

KEY POINTS

- HBeAg-positive and HBeAg-negative patients with persistently elevated HBV DNA levels >20,000 IU/mL and ALT >2x ULN (based on AASLD current treatment guidelines).
- Patients with clinically apparent cirrhosis and detectable HBV DNA regardless of ALT do not require liver biopsy for a treatment decision (based on EASL treatment guidelines).
- HBeAg positive and HBeAg negative hepatitis with HBV DNA levels greater than 20,000 IU/mL and 2000 IU/mL, respectively, and elevated AL (suggested by Keeffe algorithm).
- Patients at high risk for HCC and disease progression (ie, family history of HCC; HCV, HDV, HIV coinfection; Genotype C, high viral load) do not require liver biopsy for a treatment decision.
- Patients with contraindications for liver biopsy.

EXPERT OPINION

Is Liver Biopsy a Prerequisite to Impact on the Natural History of Hepatitis B?

by Robert Perrillo, MD

The preceding discussions by Drs. Nazario and Landaverde remind us that uniform agreement is lacking on whether a liver biopsy is necessary before finalizing a decision to treat HBV. As pointed out by Dr. Nazario, the most relevant histologic finding is the degree of fibrosis, but serum markers for this have not fulfilled the promise that they once were hoped to have. Fibroscan appears to be a promising future tool, but availability may prove to be limited by requirement for specialized expertise. Also, as pointed out by Dr. Nazario, there are several patient factors that increase liver stiffness other than fibrosis.[6-8] Perhaps the most relevant one for HBV is that the degree of stiffness is affected by the level of inflammation in the liver. A significant correlation has been shown between Fibroscan signal and ALT levels, and fluctuations in measurements have been shown to parallel hepatitis flares during chronic HBV.[43]

Thus, liver biopsy still holds a place as the gold standard for determining the extent of cellular injury and fibrosis.[9] The truth, however, is that liver biopsy is often more equivalent to "highly polished brass" in clinical practice situations due primarily to inadequate sample size. Using the Metavir system to evaluate patients with hepatitis C, it has been concluded that a length of at least 25 mm is necessary to evaluate fibrosis accurately.[41] My own experience in reviewing outside slides is consistent with ter Borg and associates who found that 90% of biopsy samples are less than 20 mm in length.[44] Furthermore, I have found that the interpretations are often further compromised by obtaining a specimen with too narrow a needle (eg, 18 mm).

Reliability of Alanine Aminotransferase and Hepatitis B Virus DNA Thresholds for Estimating Degree of Liver Injury

Dr. Landaverde asserts that the decision to treat can be made on ALT and HBV DNA levels, as recommended in the published practice guidelines of the AASLD, EASL, and Asian Pacific Association for the Study of the Liver (APASL).[12,18,19] All 3 management guidelines recognize that liver biopsy can be useful, but the AASLD Practice Guidelines is the only one to state that liver biopsy is generally not required provided certain ALT and HBV DNA limits are reached. Unfortunately, the reliance on a certain level of ALT (greater than twice the upper limit) can lead to the perception that this accurately identifies individuals with moderate to severe hepatitis. One problem with using these ALT criteria, however, is that they reflect a snapshot in time and do not convey the potential for progression in such a longstanding and dynamic disease as chronic HBV. Another problem is that a strong correlation between ALT and extent of fibrosis or necroinflammatory response has never been demonstrated for chronic HBV. For example, early studies with alpha interferon demonstrated that biopsies from individuals with ALT values 2 to 3 times the upper limit of normal often had relatively modest histologic activity and fibrosis scores; most of these patients acquired their disease in adult life and, as a result, the disease duration was relatively short, being measured in years rather than decades.[45,46] Nor has the converse been shown; as pointed out by Dr. Nazario, individuals who acquire their infection early in life may have minimal elevation or even high normal ALT and yet significant inflammation and fibrosis can be present on biopsy. The reason for this remains speculative, but it seems plausible that mild immune clearance and secondary inflammation over several decades can result in significant injury without reaching ALT levels that warrant treatment, according to the Practice Guidelines. In other words, disease duration and disease intensity are both important for accumulative liver damage. Thus, it is not surprising that in one follow up study of predominantly Asian HBsAg carriers, as many as 30% of middle age to older individuals dying of chronic HBV did not meet ALT criteria set forth in the current Practice Guidelines.[47] In a second study, inflammatory activity in explants of patients transplanted for HBV-related cirrhosis was shown not to correlate with ALT or HBV DNA level.[48]

The Need for Liver Biopsy Should Depend on the Aim of Therapy

Many hepatologists primarily focus on categorizing the extent of necroinflammatory changes and degree of fibrosis when making decisions about treatment. This practice is necessary so that physicians do not unwittingly place patients with minimal liver injury on expensive and potentially long-term care options. The development of short-term treatments that could permanently suppress viral replication in the majority of patients would place less demand on the physician for this type of selection and would make liver biopsy less relevant. In the current clinical environment, however, liver biopsy has more advantages than disadvantages.

During the past 5 years, several Asian natural history studies involving large populations of HBsAg carriers followed for more than 10 years have demonstrated that the best predictor for the risk of cirrhosis and hepatocellular carcinoma is the serum HBV DNA level.[36,49-51] In the Risk Evaluation of Viral Load Elevation and Associated Liver Disease (REVEAL) study, the sequential incidence rates of chronic hepatitis, cirrhosis, and hepatocellular carcinoma in 2100 HBsAg carriers with persistently normal ALT were shown to be strongly associated with persistence of serum HBV DNA levels in excess of 2000 IU/mL until the last point of follow up.[52] Taken together, these natural history studies provide compelling evidence that the duration and level of viral replication both interact to cause disease progression and complications. Moreover, the subgroup analysis from the REVEAL study strongly suggests that these events cannot be predicted by ALT but instead by unchanging viral replication. It is important to consider that two-thirds of the patients entering the REVEAL study were over the age of 40, 85% were HBeAg-negative, and 94% had ALT levels less than 45 IU at entry.[36] These features are reminiscent of those described in the studies alluded to by Dr. Nazario in which significant liver injury was detected despite minimally elevated or even normal ALT.[22-25]

Chronic HBV is the most common cause of HCC in the world today, and it has been estimated that 30% of cases occur in patients who do not have cirrhosis.[53] One potential pathogenetic mechanism for hepatocellular carcinoma is viral genetic integration at critical sites within the cellular genome.[54] It can be anticipated, therefore, that the higher the level of viral replication, the greater the statistical likelihood that this type of intracellular event would occur. It has already been demonstrated that antiviral therapy can forestall disease progression and interrupt the pathway leading to hepatocellular carcinoma in a large treatment cohort of Asian HBsAg carriers.[42] Thus, if the aim of treatment is to prevent future complications such as cirrhosis and liver cancer, the extent of liver injury becomes less relevant than sustained high level viral replication and, correspondingly, so does liver biopsy.

Like tobacco, HBV is a class I carcinogen. The most effective way to reduce the risk of future complications from any carcinogen is to limit exposure. For HBV, this means permanent suppression of viral replication, equivalent to permanent cessation of smoking after decades of exposure. However, just as late cessation of smoking does not fully protect against complications such as emphysema and lung cancer, late clearance of HBeAg and suppression of active viral replication has been associated with a greater chance of cirrhosis, liver failure, and liver cancer.[55]

What we have learned about the natural history and treatment of HBV over the past several years begs the question then as to whether we should consider a new treatment paradigm of maintenance antiviral therapy to prevent complications in actively viremic middle aged or older patients with early life acquisition of HBV. I believe that the answer to this is yes, because we finally have drugs that can make a difference and can be given safely long-term without major concerns about drug resistance. My personal philosophy, therefore, has gradually shifted toward offering long-term oral antiviral therapy to HBeAg-positive or negative HBsAg carriers over the age of 45 who have HBV DNA levels greater than 20,000 IU/mL irrespective of ALT level. The aim of treatment is to maintain viral DNA levels as low as possible, and it really does not matter if fibrosis is minimal or extensive in these patients. When following this treatment paradigm, biopsy is not really necessary.

References

1. Bottero J, Lacombe K, Guechot J, et al. Performance of 11 biomarkers for liver fibrosis assessment in HIV/HBV co-infected patients. *J Hepatol.* 2009;50(6):1074-1083.
2. Patel K, Lajoie A, Heaton S, et al. Clinical use of hyaluronic acid as a predictor of fibrosis change in hepatitis C. *J Gastroenterol Hepatol.* 2003;18(3):253-257.
3. Kim Y, Kim SU, Ahn SH, et al. Usefulness of Fibroscan for detection of early compensated liver cirrhosis in chronic hepatitis B. *Dig Dis Sci.* 2009;54(8):1758-1763.
4. Fung J, Lai CL, Chan SC, et al. Correlation of liver stiffness and histological features in healthy persons and in patients with occult hepatitis B, chronic active hepatitis B, or hepatitis B cirrhosis. *Am J Gastroenterol.* 2010;105(5):1116-1122.
5. Fraquelli M, Rigamonti C, Casazza G, et al. Reproducibility of transient elastography in the evaluation of liver fibrosis in patients with chronic liver disease. *Gut.* 2007;56:968-973.
6. Bonino F, Arena U, Brunetto MR, et al. Liver stiffness, a non-invasive marker of liver disease: a core study group report. *Antivir Ther.* 2010;15(S3):69-78.
7. Sagir A, Erhardt A, Schmitt M, et al. Transient elastography is unreliable for detection of cirrhosis in patients with acute liver damage. *Hepatology.* 2008;47:592-595.
8. Castera L, Foucher J, Bernard PH, et al. Pitfalls of liver stiffness measurement: a 5-year prospective study of 13,369 examinations. *Hepatology.* 2010;51:828-835.
9. Mani H, Kleiner DE. Liver biopsy findings in chronic hepatitis B. *Hepatology.* 2009;49(Suppl):S61-S71.
10. Zoulim F, Perrillo R. Hepatitis B: reflections on the current approach to antiviral therapy. *J Hepatol.* 2008;48(Suppl):S2-S19.
11. Bonino F, Brunetto MR. Chronic hepatitis B e antigen (HBeAg) negative, anti-HBe-positive hepatitis B: an overview. *J Hepatol.* 2003;39(Suppl):S160-163.
12. Lok ASF, McMahon BJ. AASLD practice guidelines. Chronic hepatitis B: update 2009. *Hepatology.* 2009;50:1-36.
13. Zarski JP, Bohn B, Bastie A, et al. Characteristics of patients with dual infection by hepatitis B and C viruses. *J Hepatol.* 1998;28:27-33.
14. Thio CL. Hepatitis B and human immunodeficiency virus infection. *Hepatology.* 2009;49(Suppl):S138-S145.
15. Heidrich B, Deterding K, Tillmann HL, et al. Virological and clinical characteristics of delta hepatitis in Central Europe. *J Viral Hepatol.* 2009;16:883-894.
16. Soriano V, Vispo E, Labarga P, et al. Viral hepatitis and HIV coinfection. *Antivir Res.* 2010;85:303-315.
17. Mendes-Corrêa M, Núñez M. Management of HIV and hepatitis virus coinfection. *Expert Opin Pharmacother.* 2010;11(15):2497-2516.
18. EASL Clinical practice guidelines: management of chronic hepatitis B. European Association for the Study of the Liver. *J Hepatol.* 2009;50:227-242.
19. Liaw Y-F, Leung N, Guan R, et al. Asian-Pacific consensus statement of the management of chronic hepatitis B: a 2005 update. *Liver Int.* 2005;25:472-489.
20. Keefe EB, Dieterich DT, Han SHB, et al. A treatment algorithm for the management of chronic HBV infection in the United States: 2008 update. *Clin Gastroenterol Hepatol.* 2008;6:1315-1341.
21. Tsang PS, Trinh H, Garcia RT, et al. Significant prevalence of histologic disease in patients with chronic hepatitis B and mildly elevated serum alanine aminotransferase levels. *Clin Gastroenterol Hepatol.* 2008;6:569-574.
22. Kumar M, Sarin SK, Hissar S, et al. Virologic and histologic features of chronic HBV-infected asymptomatic patients with persistently normal ALT. *Gastroenterology.* 2008;134:1376-1384.
23. Lai M, Hyatt BJ, Nasser I, et al. The clinical significance of persistently normal ALT in chronic hepatitis B infection. *J Hepatol.* 2007;47:760-767.
24. Hu K, Schiff ER, Kowdley KV, et al. Histologic evidence of active liver injury in chronic hepatitis B patients with normal range or minimally elevated alanine aminotransferase levels. *J Clin Gastroenterol.* 2010;44:510-516.
25. Wang CC, Lim LY, Deubner H, Tapia K, et al. Factors predictive of significant hepatic fibrosis in adults with chronic hepatitis B and normal serum ALT. *J Clin Gastroenterol.* 2008;42:820-826.

26. Sull JW, Yun JE, Lee SY, et al. Body mass index and serum aminotransferase levels in Korean men and women. *J Clin Gastroenterol.* 2009;43:869-875.

27. Adams LA, Knuiman NW, Divitini ML, Olynyk JK. Body mass index is a stronger predictor of alanine aminotransferase levels than alcohol consumption. *J Gastroenterol Hepatol.* 2008;23:1089-1093.

28. Lee JK, Shim JH, Lee HC, et al. Estimation of the healthy upper limits for serum alanine aminotransferase in Asian populations with normal liver histology. *Hepatology.* 2010;51:1577-1583.

29. Prati D, Taioli E, Zanella A, et al. Updated definitions of healthy ranges for serum alanine aminotransferases levels. *Ann Intern Med.* 2002;137:1-9.

30. Donato F, Gelatti U, Chiesa R, et al. A case-control study on family history of liver cancer as a risk factor for hepatocellular carcinoma in North Italy. Brescia HCC Study. *Cancer Causes Control.* 1999;10:417-421.

31. Hassan MM, Spitz MR, Thomas MB, et al. The association of family history of liver cancer with hepatocellular carcinoma: a case-control study in the United States. *J Hepatol.* 2009;50:334-341.

32. Cho LY, Yang JJ, Ko KP, et al. Coinfection of hepatitis B and C viruses and risk of hepatocellular carcinoma: systematic review and meta-analysis. *Intl J Cancer.* 2011;128(1):176-184.

33. Fattovich G. Natural history and prognosis of hepatitis B. *Semin Liver Dis.* 2003;23:47-58.

34. Yim HJ, Lok AS. Natural history of chronic HBV infection: what we knew in 1981 and what we know in 2005. *Hepatology.* 2006;43(Suppl):S173-S181.

35. Tong MJ, Blatt LM, Kao JH, et al. Basal core promoter T1762/A1764 and precore A1896 mutations in hepatitis B surface antigen-positive hepatocellular carcinoma: a comparison with chronic carriers. *Liver Int.* 2007;27:1356-1363.

36. Chen CJ, Yang HI, Su J, et al. Risk of hepatocellular carcinoma across a biological gradient of serum HBV DNA level. *JAMA.* 2006;295:65-73.

37. Seeff LB, Everson GT, Morgan TR, et al. Complication rate of percutaneous liver biopsies among persons with advanced chronic liver disease in the HALT-C trial. *Clin Gastroenterol Hepatol.* 2010;8(10):877-883.

38. Rockey DC, Caldwell SH, Goodman ZD, et al. Liver biopsy. *Hepatology.* 2009;49(3):1017-1044.

39. Bravo AA, Sheth SG, Chopra S. Liver biopsy. *N Engl J Med.* 2001;344:495-500.

40. Schiano TD, Azeem S, Bodian C, et al. Importance of specimen size in accurate needle liver biopsy evaluation of patients with chronic hepatitis C. *Clin Gastroenterol Hepatol.* 2005;3:930-935.

41. Colloredo G, Guido M, Sonzogni A, et al. Impact of liver biopsy size on histological evaluation of chronic viral hepatitis: the smaller the sample, the milder the disease. *J Hepatol.* 2003;39:239-244.

42. Liaw YF, Sung JJ, Chow WC, et al. Lamivudine for patients with chronic hepatitis B and advanced liver disease. *N Engl J Med.* 2004;351:1521-1531.

43. Coco B, Oliveri F, Maina AM, et al. Transient elastography: a new surrogate marker of liver fibrosis influenced by major changes of transaminases. *J Viral Hepatol.* 2007;14:360-369.

44. ter Borg F, ten Kate FJW, Cuypers HTM, et al. A survey of liver pathology in needle biopsies from HBsAg and anti-HBe positive individuals. *J Clin Pathol.* 2000;53:541-548.

45. Perrillo RP, Schiff Er, Davis GL, et al. A randomized, controlled trial of interferon alfa-2b alone and after prednisone withdrawal for the treatment of chronic hepatitis B. The Hepatitis Interventional Therapy Group. *N Engl J Med.* 1990;323:295-301.

46. Lau D-T-Y, Everhart J, Kleiner DE, et al. Long-term follow up of patients with chronic hepatitis B treated with interferon alfa. *Gastroenterology.* 1997;113:1660-1667.

47. Tong MJ, Hsien C, Hsu L, et al. Treatment recommendations for chronic hepatitis B: an evaluation of current guidelines based on a natural history study in the United States. *Hepatology.* 2008;48:1070-1078.

48. Sigal SH, Aftab A, Ivanov K, et al. Histopathology and clinical correlates of end-stage hepatitis B cirrhosis: a possible mechanism to explain the response to antiviral therapy. *Liver Transplantation.* 2005;11:82-88.

49. Iloeje UH, Yang H-I, Su J, et al. Predicting cirrhosis based on the level of circulating hepatitis B viral load. *Gastroenterology.* 2006;130:678-686.

50. Yu M-W, Yeh S-H, Chen P-J, et al. HBV genotype and HBV DNA level and hepatocellular carcinoma: a prospective study in men. *J Natl Cancer Inst.* 2005;97:265-272.

51. Yuen M-F, Yuan H-J, Wong D K-H, et al. Determinants for chronic hepatitis B in Asians: therapeutic implications. *Gut.* 2005;54:1610-1614.

52. Chen JD, Yang HL, Iloeje UH, et al. Liver disease progression in chronic hepatitis B infected persons with normal serum alanine aminotransferase levels: update from the R.E.V.E.A.L.–HBV study group. *J Hepatol.* 2008;48(Suppl):S240.

53. Di Bisceglie AM. Hepatitis B and hepatocellular carcinoma. *Hepatology.* 2009;49(Suppl):S56-S60.

54. Blum HE, Moradpour DD. Viral pathogenesis of hepatocellular carcinoma. *J Gastroenterol Hepatol.* 2002;17(Suppl):S413-S420.

55. Chu C-M, Liaw Y-F. Chronic HBV infection acquired in childhood: special emphasis on prognostic and therapeutic implication of delayed HBeAg seroconversion. *J Viral Hepatol.* 2007;14:147-152.

Should the Decompensated Hepatitis C Cirrhotic Be Treated With Antiviral Therapy?

Payam Afshar, MD; Jeffrey Weissman, MD; and Paul J. Pockros, MD

The use of pegylated interferon and ribavirin therapy in patients with decompensated liver disease due to chronic hepatitis C is a high-risk, low-reward gamble. Most patients treated in such a manner do not complete their therapy and thus do not achieve an SVR. Some of these patients experience severe complications resulting in hospitalization or death. However, the benefit to those few who are able to achieve a sustained virologic response (SVR) cannot be understated. Those patients do not reinfect the allograft after liver transplantation, thus avoiding recurrent post-transplant liver damage. And some of these patients may even avoid transplantation altogether. These life-and-death issues make this topic a timely controversy in hepatology.

POINT

Treating Decompensated Hepatitis C Cirrhotics With Antiviral Therapy May Be Appropriate Under Selected Conditions

by Payam Afshar, MD

Based on the current United Network for Organ Sharing (UNOS) data, approximately 90% of the hepatitis C virus (HCV)-related cirrhosis patients actively listed for organ transplantation in the United States have a MELD score of <18.[1] The majority of these patients listed have

Jensen D.
Controversies in Hepatology: The Experts Analyze Both Sides (pp 43-50)
© 2011 SLACK Incorporated

Table 5-1.

POPULATION OF DECOMPENSATED HEPATITIS C VIRUS-RELATED CIRRHOSIS TO CONSIDER FOR ANTIVIRAL THERAPY
■ MELD score <18 or CTP score <7 (not advised for MELD score >25 or CTP score >11).
■ HCV genotypes 2 and 3.
■ Institution of antiviral therapy administration should be done at a liver transplant center and patient should be listed for transplantation prior to therapy.

experienced at least 1 decompensation event, such as ascites, spontaneous bacterial peritonitis, hepatic encephalopathy, or bleeding esophageal varices. The American Association for the Study of Liver Diseases (AASLD) guidelines for treatment of chronic hepatitis C states that there are clear indications to treat patients with compensated HCV-related cirrhosis.[2] However, the guidelines do not recommend treatment of decompensated cirrhosis, primarily because there is sparse published information to support the safe use of pegylated interferons and ribavirin in the decompensated HCV cirrhotic.

The importance of identifying the safety of antiviral therapy in this specific patient population is paramount because once transplanted, graft and patient survival in this population is significantly lower in comparison to patients who undergo liver transplantation for other causes.[3] Despite the importance of addressing treatment in this large patient population, limited data have been published since 2002 concerning the use of interferon-based therapy. Based on the limited literature that is available, we are recommending treatment of a select population of decompensated HCV-related cirrhotics awaiting liver transplantation (Table 5-1).

Goals of Therapy in the Decompensated Hepatitis C Virus Cirrhotic

There are 2 goals to antiviral therapy in the HCV cirrhotic listed for liver transplantation. The first is to achieve SVR in hopes of eradicating the virus and preventing recurrence in the graft. The second, if SVR is not achieved, is to decrease viral load to improve the length of graft survival.

Based on collected data of 210 patients with decompensated HCV-cirrhosis, the median SVR achieved was 16.6% (range 7% to 30%) for genotypes 1 and 4, and 47% (range 44% to 50%) for genotypes 2 and 3.[4-6] Everson et al[4] reported 15 patients who achieved SVR with decompensated cirrhosis that later underwent liver transplantation. Eighty percent of these patients maintained their HCV-RNA negative status at 6 months of follow-up post-transplantation.

If SVR cannot be obtained, an alternative goal of therapy is to decrease viral load and graft survival. This benefit can be seen in patients with the option of live donor liver transplantation (LDLT) or those likely to undergo liver transplantation within 4 months of antiviral therapy initiation. The National Institute of Diabetes and Digestive and Kidney Diseases (NIDDK) Liver Transplant Database reported that patients with lower levels of hepatitis C viremia (<1 x 106 viral copies/mL) before liver transplantation had improved 1- and 5-year patient survival of 94% and 83%, respectively, compared to those with higher levels of viremia with 1- and 5-year survival of 83% and 57%, respectively.[7] This establishes some scientific basis for lowering pretransplant viral load as a therapeutic goal.

Population to Treat Among the Decompensated Hepatitis C Virus Cirrhotic

Careful selection of patients with decompensated HCV-cirrhosis to initiate antiviral therapy is critical because of the hematologic side effects to interferon and ribavirin therapy. In the patient with end-stage liver disease, these often result in dose reductions, cessation of therapy, and sometimes morbidity and mortality. Furthermore, the SVR rates of 40% to 50% in genotype 1, 55% to 70% in genotype 4, and 80% in genotypes 2 and 3 seen in noncirrhotic HCV patients are not seen in the cirrhotic patient population. Iacobellis et al published the recent data on combined therapy of pegylated interferon and ribavirin.[5] All of the patients had decompensated HCV cirrhosis with the majority of the patients comprising Child-Pugh classes B and C with a mean MELD score of 14.2 + 2.7. SVR rates of only 7.0% were noted in those with genotype 1 while 43.5% were noted in those few cases with genotypes 2 and 3. Based on univariate analysis, genotype was the only significant factor related with viral clearance. Based on these findings, we recommend that interferon therapy should be offered to decompensated HCV cirrhotics with genotypes 2 or 3 awaiting transplantation with low MELD scores. In contrast, consideration of treatment in those with genotype 1 should be more selective as response rates have shown to be significantly lower.

Safety of Therapy

The side effects of therapy and pre-existing cytopenias in the decompensated HCV-cirrhosis population limit the standard dosing regimen of interferon and ribavirin. Everson studied a novel approach to therapy, referred to as Low Accelerating Dosage Regimen (LADR), in HCV cirrhotics, the majority of which experienced at least one decompensating event.[8] The rationale for slow escalation of antiviral therapy was to enhance tolerance in hopes of clearance or suppression of viral activity prior to time of liver transplantation. Of 124 patients in the study, 15 developed 22 complications (12%), the majority of which were related to underlying liver decompensation such as encephalopathy and ascites. Only 2 patients experienced a treatment-associated death in the study. In contrast to the aforementioned study, 3 other single-center trials have all found much higher mortality rates.[6,9,10] Furthermore, the comparison of adverse events amongst untreated versus treated patients with antiviral therapy were only analyzed in the Iacobellis study[5] which showed a significant decrease in ascites, encephalopathy, bleeding, and hepatocellular carcinoma in treated patients, regardless of viral clearance. Also, deaths were more frequent in controls than those who were treated regardless if SVR was obtained.[5] These data are encouraging; however, the rates of infection were higher in the treatment group than the control arm.

KEY POINTS

- SVR can be obtained in up to 16% of genotype 1 and up to 47% of genotype 2/3 patients with decompensated cirrhosis with MELD scores <15.

- Patients with lower levels of hepatitis C viremia (<1 x 106 viral copies/mL) before liver transplantation had improved 1- and 5-year patient survival.

- The rationale for slow escalation of antiviral therapy (LADR) is to enhance tolerance in hopes of clearance or suppression of viral activity prior to liver transplantation.

- The increased morbidity and mortality related to infection from LADR therapy must be compared to the risks of complications and death in the untreated population.

Treating Decompensated Hepatitis C Cirrhotics With Antiviral Therapy Should Not Be Undertaken

by Jeffrey Weissman, MD

Interferon-based antiviral therapy in compensated hepatitis C-related cirrhosis has been shown to be safe and effective in virus eradication. The goal of therapy is pretransplant virus eradication with reduced post-transplant hepatitis C-related disease recurrence and to possibly delay or avoid the need for liver transplantation. Although the AASLD has endorsed low-dose antiviral therapy for patients with mild hepatic decompensation awaiting liver transplantation, significant questions remain regarding both treatment efficacy and safety.[2]

Trials addressing interferon-based therapy efficacy have shown some promise in patients with low MELD scores and genotypes 2 and 3 infection but have been disappointing in genotype 1, the predominant genotype in North America (Table 5-2).[4-6,8] Thomas et al used a high-dose interferon regimen, yielding an overall 60% rate of undetectable virus RNA prior to transplant. However, 67% of these pretransplant responders showed post-transplant recurrence. The mean MELD score for responders was 13, with only 2 participants with MELD scores greater than 15 at enrollment, thus limiting the therapy to relatively less ill patients.

Iacobellis showed 43% SVR rates in genotype 2 and 3 patients and only 7% SVR in genotype 1 and 4 patients.[5] Using a low accelerating dose regimen, Everson showed a 50% SVR in genotype 2 and 3 patients, but only a 13% SVR in genotype 1 patients.[8] The mean MELD score in Everson's trials was 11, again limiting therapy to those patients who were less ill. In Barcelona, Forns et al showed an overall 30% response rate to therapy pretransplantation, with one-third showing post-transplant recurrence.[9] Thus, treatment response rates are low, particularly so in genotype 1 patients, with significant post-transplant recurrence.

Interferon-based therapy also poses significant safety risks in this clinically vulnerable population. Crippin examined 15 patients with mean Child-Pugh score 11.9 undergoing interferon therapy with or without ribavirin, finding 23 adverse events, 20 serious adverse events, and 1 death.[10] Forns reported treatment cessation of an interferon/ribavirin regimen in 20% of patients and treatment interruption in an additional 13%, with 2 cases of sepsis and 60% of patients experiencing neutropenia.[9] Everson reported 23 adverse events affecting 15 of 124 patients enrolled, with 4 patient deaths, 2 of which the authors felt may have been treatment-related.[8] Iacobellis reported an increased risk of infection (odds ratio [OR] 2.43, CI 1.02 to 5.77), severe infection (2.95 OR, CI 0.9 to 9.3) and infection-related death (OR 1.97, CI 0.40 to 9.51) in interferon/ribavirin-treated patients versus untreated controls.[5] Serious adverse events severely limit the applicability of interferon-based therapy in decompensated cirrhosis.

Although pretransplantation treatment aimed at prolonging time to transplant and minimizing post-transplant disease recurrence is an important goal, data do not yet show interferon-based regimens to be generally effective, notably so in genotype 1 patients. Further, significant adverse events, ranging from cytopenias to infection to death are frequent, treatment limiting, and unwarranted. These risks are particularly unacceptable in patients with the highest MELD scores who are most susceptible to complications and have shorter wait times to transplant. Viral resistance in those unable to complete therapy pretransplant may also complicate post-transplant therapy. Data do not support pretransplant treatment of hepatitis C virus in decompensated cirrhotics.

Table 5-2.

STUDY ADVERSE EFFECTS

STUDY	TEKIN et al (2008)	CRIPPIN et al (2002)	FORNS et al (2003)	EVERSON et al (2005)	THOMAS et al (2003)	IACOBELLIS et al (2006)
DRUG REGIMEN	PEG-INF alfa 2a plus ribavirin	INF alfa 2b with or without ribavirin	INF alfa 2b plus ribavirin	INF alfa 2b or PEG-INF alfa 2b plus ribavirin	INF alfa 2b	PEG-INF alfa 2b
NUMBER TREATED	20	15	30	124	20	66
MELD	NR	NR	NR	11.0 +/- 3.7	16.7 +/- 2.4	14.2 +/- 2.7 (24.3% >18)
CHILD-PUGH SCORE	30% A 70% B	Mean 11.9 +/- 1.2	50% A 43% B 7% C	7.4 +/- 2.3	10.4 +/- 0.7	6% A 71% B 23% C
OVERALL AE	NR	23	NR	23	NR	45
DEATH	0	1	0	4 (2 study related)	0	5
MOST COMMON AE	PSE, HCC (10%)	Thrombocytopenia (50%)	Neutropenia (60%)	PSE	NR	Infection

MELD = Model for End-Stage Liver Disease; INF = interferon; PEG = pegylated; NR = not reported; PSE = portosystemic encephalopathy; HCC = hepatocellular carcinoma

KEY POINTS

- SVR can be obtained in patients with decompensated cirrhosis but these are usually genotype 2/3 patients with MELD scores <11.
- Results with genotype 1 patients or those with higher MELD scores are poor.
- Interferon-based therapy also poses significant safety risks in this population, especially for increased risk of infection (OR 2.43), severe infection (OR 2.95) and infection-related death (OR 1.97).
- Serious adverse event severely limit the applicability of interferon-based therapy in decompensated cirrhosis.

EXPERT OPINION

How Do We Adjudicate These Opposing Opinions?

by Paul J. Pockros, MD

Our opposing sides only seem to agree that treatment of the decompensated cirrhotic patient may be attempted safely in the patient with a low MELD score and genotype 2 or 3. This is certainly a rarity in our experience, as the majority of patients are genotype 1 and most have MELD scores above 15. Our authors disagree about the safety and wisdom of treating this group. One side suggests we may safely try LADR therapy, although success rates are low. The other side suggests the risk of infectious complications and/or death is too high to even consider therapy in this population, especially when the chance of SVR is low. So how do we adjudicate these opposing opinions?

There is hope, I believe, that the new direct-acting antivirals (DAAs) anticipated for approval this year will be an important addition to our therapy. Unfortunately, the current studies with DAAs have shown clearly that they must be developed in combination with pegylated interferons and ribavirin.[11] If one gives an NS3/4 protease inhibitor without interferon, then rapid emergence of resistant variants occurs, even with very potent drugs.[12] If one leaves out ribavirin, then high relapse rates occur and SVR is significantly reduced.[13]

Therefore, the limitations that have been discussed in the previous arguments will continue to apply to treatments that include DAAs for the near future. However, we anticipate shortening the duration of therapy to 24 weeks for many of the genotype 1 patients and improving the SVR rates of those seen in the genotype 2 and 3 patient groups, in all likelihood. This would clearly be an improvement over our current poor choices with this population. We have hope that interferon-free regimens will ultimately be an option for these patients, based on the early favorable data we have seen to date.[14]

The ideal option for the decompensated HCV cirrhotic would be an interferon-free regimen that also minimized ribavirin dosing to avoid the cytopenias and anemia caused by therapy. We can only hope these regimens will be effective and made available to our decompensated HCV patients sooner than later.

References

1. Wiesner RH, Sorell M, Villamil F, and the International Liver Transplantation Society Expert Panel. Report of the first International Liver Transplantation Society Expert Panel consensus conference on liver transplantation and hepatitis C. *Liver Transplantation.* 2003;9(11):S1-S9.
2. Strader DB, Wright T, Thomas DL, Seef LB. AASLD practice guideline: diagnosis, management, and treatment of hepatitis C. *Hepatology.* 2004;39:1147-1171.
3. Forman LM, Lewis JD, Berlin JA, et al. The association between hepatitis C infection and survival after liver transplantation. *Hepatology.* 2002;35:680-687.
4. Everson G. Treatment of patients with hepatitis C virus on the waiting list. *J Hepatol.* 2005;42:456-462.
5. Iacobellis A, Siciliano M, Perri, F, et al. Peginterferon alpha-2b and ribavirin in patients with hepatitis C virus and decompensated cirrhosis: a controlled study. *J Hepatol.* 2007;46:206-212.
6. Tekin F, Gunsar F, Karasu Z, et al. Safety, tolerability, and efficacy of pegylated-interferon alpha-2a plus ribavirin in HCV-related decompensated cirrhotics. *Aliment Pharmacol Ther.* 2008;27(11):1081-1085.
7. Charlton M, Seaberg E, Wiesner R, et al. Predictors of patient and graft survival following liver transplantation for hepatitis C. *Hepatology.* 1998;28:823-830.
8. Everson GT. Treatment of advanced hepatitis C with a low accelerating dosage regimen [LADR] of antiviral therapy. *Hepatology.* 2005;42:255-262.
9. Forns X. Antiviral therapy of patients with decompensated cirrhosis to prevent recurrence of hepatitis C after liver transplantation. *J Hepatol.* 2003;39:389-396.
10. Crippin JS. A pilot study of the tolerability and efficacy of antiviral therapy in hepatitis C virus-infected patients awaiting liver transplantation. *Liver Transpl.* 2002;8:350-355.
11. Pockros PJ. New direct acting antivirals (DAAs) in development for HCV infection. *Ther Adv Gastroenterol.* 2010;3:191-202.
12. Pawlotsky JM, Chevaliez S, McHutchison JG. The hepatitis C virus life cycle as a target for new antiviral therapies. *Gastroenterology.* 2007;132:1979-1998.
13. Hezode C, Forestier N, Dusheiko G, et al. Telaprevir and peginterferon with or without ribavirin for chronic HCV infection. *N Engl J Med.* 2009;360:1839-1850.
14. Gane EJ, Roberts SK, Stedman C, et al. Potent antiviral activity with a nucleoside polymerase (R7128) and protease (R7227/ITMN-191) inhibitor combination in HCV genotype 1: initial safety, pharmacokinetics, and virologic results from INFORM-1. *J Hepatol.* 2009;50(Suppl):S380.

SHOULD HEPATITIS C BE TREATED IN PATIENTS WITH CHRONIC KIDNEY DISEASE PRIOR TO KIDNEY TRANSPLANT?

Andres F. Carrion, MD; Seth N. Sclair, MD; and Paul Martin, MD

The management of hepatitis C virus (HCV) in renal transplant candidates remains an area of debate as HCV infection clearly leads to diminished graft and patient survivals. Compounding this issue is the poorer tolerance of interferon-based regimens in patients with chronic kidney disease due to associated morbidities, including anemia, although successful therapy can prevent graft injury due to HCV as well as progression of liver disease.

POINT

Hepatitis C Should Be Treated in Patients With End-Stage Renal Disease Prior to Kidney Transplant

by Andres F. Carrion, MD

Chronic liver disease is the fourth most common cause of death following renal transplantation, with HCV being the most frequent etiology. Interferon-based therapy is contraindicated after renal transplantation because of a high risk of allograft rejection. Therefore, current practice guidelines advocate treating transplant candidates with chronic kidney disease (CKD) prior to transplantation.[1,2]

Jensen D.
Controversies in Hepatology: The Experts Analyze Both Sides (pp 51-60)
© 2011 SLACK Incorporated

Hepatitis C Virus Infection and Patient and Renal Allograft Survival

HCV infection adversely affects patient and graft survival following renal transplantation. For instance, 8 reports comparing outcomes between HCV-positive and HCV-negative renal transplant recipients were summarized in a meta-analysis. The pooled estimates for relative risk (RR) were 1.79 (95% CI, 1.57 to 2.03) for patient death and 1.56 (95% CI, 1.35 to 1.80) for graft failure.[3] Earlier studies suggest that the increased mortality and graft failure in HCV-positive compared to HCV-negative renal transplant recipients diminished only long-term survival (ie, 10 years or more)[4]; however, more recent data from a large national registry have shown that significant differences can also be detected even with shorter follow-up intervals (ie, 4 years).[5] The higher mortality in HCV-positive patients is predominantly related to a higher incidence of liver cirrhosis and hepatocellular carcinoma. Data suggest that CKD patients who do not receive pretransplant interferon are at increased risk of developing hepatic dysfunction following renal transplantation (odds ratio [OR] 11.7, $P = 0.003$).[6]

Comorbid Conditions Associated With Hepatitis C Virus Following Renal Transplantation

Other important complications implicated in decreased patient and graft survival rates in HCV-positive renal transplant recipients include allograft nephropathy, new-onset diabetes after transplantation (NODAT), and a higher frequency of sepsis.[7,8] HCV-positive patients also have a higher incidence of proteinuria following renal transplantation compared to HCV-negative controls (RR = 5.36 [95% CI, 2.49 to 11])[9] along with an increased risk of recurrence of the original renal disease.[10] The incidence of de novo glomerulonephritis following renal transplantation varies significantly depending on the recipient's HCV status (34% to 6.6% for HCV-positive and HCV-negative patients, respectively).[11] Results from a small, uncontrolled clinical trial show that pretransplant interferon therapy decreases the incidence of de novo glomerulonephritis to 7%. None of the patients who achieved sustained virologic response (SVR) (67%) developed this complication.[12] The prognosis of de novo glomerulonephritis is worse in HCV-positive than in HCV-negative renal transplant recipients, and HCV infection also increases the risk of allograft failure and return to dialysis.[13] Data from a retrospective study show that pretransplant treatment with standard interferon may result in a 50% reduction of acute graft rejection; however, SVR rates were not reported.[14] HCV infection is also associated with insulin resistance, and HCV-positive renal transplant recipients have a 3- to 5-fold higher incidence of NODAT than HCV-negative controls (pooled OR = 3.97 [95% CI, 1.83 to 8.61]).[15] Furthermore, NODAT increases all-cause mortality and the incidence of major cardiovascular events (ie, cardiac death or nonfatal acute myocardial infarction) by 3-fold, hence significantly reducing patient survival compared to nondiabetic post-transplant patients (20% to 37%, respectively, after 8 years of follow-up).[16] Pretransplant therapy with standard interferon may decrease the prevalence of NODAT from 25% to 7%; however, it is unclear if the benefit reflects fewer episodes of acute graft rejection requiring glucocorticoids or if it is directly associated with virological response; SVR rates were not reported and subgroup analyses were not done.[14]

Recommendations for Anti-Hepatitis C Virus Therapy Before Renal Transplantation

Current practice guidelines endorse consideration of anti-HCV therapy for CKD patients who are candidates for renal transplantation and have an estimated survival of at least 5 years; nonetheless, patient-specific characteristics must be considered in the risk-benefit assessment. The guidelines recommend treating renal transplant candidates with CKD even when the pattern of histologic injury does not meet the recommended degree of hepatic fibrosis to qualify for therapy in the general population (ie, a Metavir score ≥2 and an Ishak-Knodell score ≥3).[1] For HCV-infected patients undergoing hemodialysis, monotherapy with standard interferon alpha-2a or alpha-2b at a dose of 3 million units subcutaneously 3 times a week is currently the recommended regimen. Treatment with this drug has resulted in a pooled SVR of 39% and a drop-out rate of 19%.[17] Reduced dose pegylated interferon alpha-2a (135 µg/week) or alpha-2b (1 µg/kg/week) may also be used in renal transplant candidates[2]; however, a recent meta-analysis showed that monotherapy with these drugs results in a slightly lower SVR (33%) and higher drop-out rates (23%) compared with standard interferon.[18] Furthermore, management of adverse reactions may be less complicated with standard interferon because of its shorter half-life and lesser pharmacokinetic variation associated with hemodialysis.[19] Ribavirin is generally not recommended for patients with glomerular filtration rates less than 50 mL/minute/1.73 m[2]; nonetheless, data from small, uncontrolled trials using this drug in combination with interferon in CKD patients undergoing hemodialysis have shown encouraging results with either the administration of fixed low-doses of ribavirin or with adjustments in the dose to target specific plasma ribavirin concentrations (10 to 15 µmol/L) to prevent hemoglobin levels to decrease below preset values.[20-23] It should be noted, though, that this therapeutic approach requires aggressive concomitant growth factor support to decrease the incidence of severe hemolytic anemia associated with ribavirin toxicity in hemodialysis patients but it may result in an increased number of patients achieving SVR.

KEY POINTS

- HCV-positive renal transplant recipients exhibit reduced patient and graft survival rates.
- De novo glomerulonephritis is five times more common in HCV-positive versus HCV-negative transplant recipients.
- Pre-renal transplant treatment for HCV significantly decreases the incidence of de novo glomerulonephritis.
- The incidence of new-onset diabetes after transplantation is 3- to 5-fold higher in HCV-positive renal transplant recipients than in HCV-negative controls.
- Monotherapy with standard interferon is the recommended therapeutic regimen for CKD patients undergoing hemodialysis.
- SVR is achieved in 39% of CKD patients undergoing hemodialysis that are treated with standard interferon.

COUNTERPOINT

Hepatitis C Should Not be Treated in Patients With Chronic Kidney Disease Prior to Kidney Transplantation

by Seth N. Sclair, MD

HCV remains prevalent among patients with CKD. For instance, rates of infection in US hemodialysis centers are as high as 14.0%[24] and in Western European countries prevalence rates are between 2.6% to 22.9%.[2,24] Hemodialysis patients infected with HCV have higher mortality rates compared to noninfected hemodialysis patients, reflecting complications of liver disease.[2,25,26] A meta-analysis by Fabrizi et al demonstrated the impact of HCV on the mortality of patients on hemodialysis with an adjusted relative risk of all-cause mortality of 1.34 (95% CI, 1.13 to 1.59) in a sample size of 11,589 patients.[27] In this analysis, liver-related causes of death (ie, hepatocellular carcinoma and cirrhosis) were found to be significantly higher in patients on maintenance hemodialysis with positive anti-HCV antibodies than dialysis patients with negative anti-HCV antibodies (RR 3.75, [95% CI, 2.02 to 6.96]), whereas the relative risk of cardiovascular-related death (RR 0.94 [95% CI, 0.76 to 1.18]) and infections (RR 1.25 [95% CI, 0.88 to 1.78]) were not found to be different in these groups.[27] However, this is not entirely consistent in the literature. Di Napoli et al[28] has demonstrated significantly higher proportions of death due to infection in the HCV group, and Kalantar-Zadeh et al[29] have shown significantly higher proportions of death due to cardiovascular disease. These latter 2 reports, however, also reflect the frequency of important comorbidities in the hemodialysis population as a whole.

The rationale for treating HCV in this patient group is clear: to halt progression of liver disease pre- and post-transplant, improve patient survival, and prevent renal graft injury due to HCV infection, as well as reduce the likelihood of post-transplant diabetes mellitus. However, there are important considerations unique to patients with advanced CKD limiting treatment of HCV in this patient group. These include the potential toxicity of antiviral therapy, low SVR rates, and poor tolerability of therapy. Therefore, treatment approaches for patients with HCV and intact renal function cannot be uncritically applied to patients with renal disease.[25]

Toxicity of Antiviral Therapy

Adverse reactions of interferon-based therapy are many and include gastrointestinal, neuropsychiatric, and influenza-like symptoms, as well as hematologic abnormalities. The latter are a particular concern in CKD patients who have a high baseline prevalence of anemia. The following side effects are reported at rates greater than 20% even in the absence of renal failure: fatigue, headache, pyrexia, myalgia, rigors, insomnia, nausea, alopecia, irritability, arthralgia, anorexia, weight loss, injection site reaction, dermatitis, and depression.[30,31] Interferon-induced depression is reported in 20% to 30% of patients, and interferon therapy frequently worsens underlying psychiatric problems. Thyroid disorders (both hypo- and hyperthyroidism) occur in 1% to 6% of patients treated with interferon. Pulmonary side effects of interferon alpha include interstitial lung disease, alveolar disease, and sarcoidosis. Interferon alpha has also been reported to cause worsening of neuropathy and retinopathy, of particular concern in patients with CKD due to diabetes mellitus.[31] In general, side effects of interferon-based therapy are more intense in the hemodialysis population, as these patients are typically older with significant comorbid conditions.[32]

Both standard and pegylated interferons suppress hematopoiesis with a reduction in hemoglobin levels.[31] Neutropenia occurs at a rate of up to 20% with pegylated interferon versus 5% in standard interferon therapy; a 21% median drop in neutrophil count has been demonstrated after just one injection of pegylated interferon. Severe neutropenia occurs at a rate of 4%. Thrombocytopenia occurs at a rate of 4% in pegylated interferon therapy and 1% in standard interferon therapy, accounting for a 10% to 50% drop in platelet counts.[30,31]

Hemolytic anemia due to ribavirin is a particular concern in patients with CKD. Since ribavirin is renally excreted and is not efficiently dialyzed, ribavirin and its metabolites accumulate.[20,30,32,33] Even in patients with normal renal function receiving standard interferon and ribavirin, there is a mean maximal decrease of 3 g/dL of hemoglobin within the first 2 to 4 weeks of therapy, and in approximately 9% of patients hemoglobin levels will fall below 10 g/dL.[30] Therefore, the major toxicity of ribavirin is poorly tolerated in patients with CKD with already high rates of baseline anemia. If ribavirin is used in this population, its dosage must be markedly reduced, hemoglobin levels must be monitored closely, and erythropoietin must be used aggressively to maintain hemoglobin levels.[32]

Low Sustained Virologic Response Rates

Patients with renal disease and HCV infection who are treated with interferon monotherapy have overall lower rates of SVR compared to patients with normal renal function receiving combination therapy. Typically this is inferred from the literature, rather than reflecting randomized trials with comparisons between these 2 groups of patients. In a meta-analysis of hemodialysis patients treated with standard interferon monotherapy, SVR was estimated as 37% overall and 30% in HCV genotype 1 patients. Similarly, in another meta-analysis, SVR was 33% overall and 26% in patients with genotype 1.[26,32,34,35] Interestingly, these SVR rates appear higher than in patients with normal renal function receiving monotherapy with standard interferon, but lower when compared to treatment with the current standard of care of pegylated interferon and ribavirin.[17] In general, overall SVR rates in combination therapy with pegylated interferon alpha-2b and alpha-2a and ribavirin are 54% and 56%, respectively, in patients with normal renal function.[2]

The literature is limited as far as investigating the role of pegylated interferon monotherapy in patients with CKD on hemodialysis. Most studies have been small with fewer than 10 patients with SVR rate reported as high as 75%.[25] However, the larger study of 78 patients conducted by Covic et al and another study of 34 patients by Tan et al with pegylated interferon alfa-2a have demonstrated SVR rates of 14.0% and 50.0%, respectively.[36,37] The frequency of adverse events in hemodialysis patients receiving monotherapy with pegylated interferon results in 30% to 50% of patients unable to complete therapy.[25] As a result of the low SVR rates and poor tolerability of pegylated interferon in hemodialysis patients, its use is not recommended in this setting.

Finally, several small, uncontrolled clinical trials have described the use of ribavirin in patients with reduced glomerular filtration rates (GFR). Bruchfeld et al and Carriero et al demonstrated SVR of 50% and 29%, respectively, when using pegylated interferon and ribavirin in hemodialysis patients.[38,39] However, the sample sizes in these studies are small (6 patients and 14 patients) and drop-out rates have been extremely high (Carriero et al reported 71.4%). Therefore, these results are not widely generalizable.

Tolerance of Therapy

Patients with CKD and on hemodialysis do not tolerate antiviral therapy as well as patients with normal renal function. HCV patients with normal renal function require premature termination of therapy at rates of 10% in pegylated interferon-based therapy and 11% in standard interferon combination therapy. Dose reductions occur at rates of 32% in pegylated interferon-based therapy and 27% in standard interferon combination therapy.[30] In comparison, drop-out rates for interferon monotherapy in the HCV and hemodialysis populations are estimated to be 19% and only 5% to 9% in HCV patients with normal renal function receiving monotherapy.[20,32]

In addition to the CKD population being generally older with more comorbid conditions, the pharmacokinetics of interferon are altered in CKD. The half-life of interferon is longer than in patients with normal renal function (9.6 hours as compared to 5.3 hours).[2,32,34] This may explain, in part, why dialysis patients have more difficulty tolerating therapy and have higher drop-out rates.

Additional Considerations

Treatment of HCV with antiviral therapy is not recommended in patients with a life expectancy of less than 5 years, and patients with HCV and CKD on hemodialysis tend to have other medical comorbidities in addition to their kidney disease with overall decreased life expectancies. Finally, treatment of HCV with interferon-based regimens in patients with CKD may preclude active listing of these patients for renal transplant, thereby delaying renal transplantation.[1,2,32] If transfusion is required for treatment–induced anemia, this may sensitize the patient and make cross-matching problematic during subsequent renal transplant.[40]

Summary

Antiviral treatment in the hemodialysis patient population with HCV infection is frequently toxic, especially when ribavirin is used. Without ribavirin, antiviral therapy is less effective and SVR is achieved at much lower rates. Finally, drop-out rates are higher in this patient group due to the difficulty involved in tolerating therapy. Patients are older with higher rates of coronary artery disease, congestive heart failure, anemia, and other comorbid conditions, thereby making these patients more susceptible to toxicities and adverse effects of antiviral therapy. This decreased tolerability of therapy results in increased drop-out rates, the discontinuation of therapy, and dose reductions. Therefore, despite the theoretical benefits of increased graft survival rates and decreased overall mortality post-renal transplantation, treatment of HCV infection in this setting is not recommended.

KEY POINTS

- The toxicities of interferon-based therapy in patients with CKD are poorly tolerated.
- The effect of hemolytic anemia due to ribavirin precludes its safe use in patients with CKD.
- SVR rates achieved with interferon monotherapy in patients with CKD are much lower than the SVR rates for patients with normal renal function receiving treatment with pegylated interferon and ribavirin.
- Studies of pegylated interferon monotherapy in hemodialysis patients have demonstrated high drop-out rates (30% to 50% of patients are unable to complete therapy).
- Studies using ribavirin in hemodialysis patients have been uncontrolled in design, small in sample size, and have demonstrated inconsistent results with high drop-out rates.

EXPERT OPINION

Hepatitis C Virus Therapy in Renal Transplant: Balancing the Risks

by Paul Martin, MD

It has been unequivocally demonstrated that HCV infection impacts survival in patients with CKD. However, given the limitations of current antiviral regimens for HCV, it is clearly impractical and of limited benefit to treat many CKD patients infected with HCV even in patients with normal renal function. Therapy is best directed toward patients with likely good long-term survival with limited comorbidities, given the high attrition rate of patients overall on chronic hemodialysis. Patients deemed to be otherwise acceptable renal transplant candidates are more robust than the dialysis population as a whole and derive benefit from renal transplant despite HCV infection.[41,42] This is the subset of CKD patients requiring renal replacement therapy who have the most to gain from successful antiviral therapy with decreased risk of graft injury due to HCV and less risk of progression of their liver disease. However, even in these patients antiviral therapy with the currently licensed regimens may be poorly tolerated. The decision to proceed to renal transplant in a viremic HCV-infected recipient should take into consideration histological severity of the liver disease, as cirrhotic patients are poor candidates for isolated renal transplant. Although direct-acting antiviral agents hold great promise in the management of HCV infection, there is no information about their use in patients with renal dysfunction and it therefore seems unlikely that treatment options for HCV in CKD will expand in the next several years. If antiviral therapy is attempted prior to renal transplant, careful attention to comorbidities, such as cardiac and retinal disease, is necessary to lessen the risk of major toxicities. Other aspects to take into consideration when determining whether to attempt therapy should include favorable genotype and lower viral load in an individual renal transplant candidate. Clearly therapy in this setting should only be undertaken by health care providers experienced in treating HCV in complex patients. An absence of response or inability to tolerate therapy should not be a reason to deny renal transplant in a patient with histologically mild HCV.

References

1. Kidney disease: improving global outcomes. KDIGO clinical practice guidelines for the prevention, diagnosis, evaluation, and treatment of hepatitis C in chronic kidney disease. *Kidney Int Suppl.* 2008;109:S1-S99.

2. Ghany MG, Strader DB, Thomas DL, et al. Diagnosis, management, and treatment of hepatitis C: an update. *Hepatology.* 2009;49:1335-1374.

3. Fabrizi F, Martin P, Dixit V, et al. Hepatitis C virus antibody status and survival after renal transplantation: meta-analysis of observational studies. *Am J Transplant.* 2005;5:1452-1461.

4. Domínguez-Gil, Morales JM. Transplantation in the patient with hepatitis C. *Transplant Int.* 2009;22:1117-1131.

5. Morales JM, Marcén R, Andres A, et al. Renal transplantation in patients with hepatitis C virus antibody: a long national experience. *NDT Plus.* 2010;3(Suppl):ii41-ii46.

6. Mahmoud IM, Sobh MA, El-Habashi AF, et al. Interferon therapy in hemodialysis patients with chronic hepatitis C: a study of tolerance, efficacy and post-transplantation course. *Nephron Clin Pract.* 2005;100:c133-c139.

7. Lee WC, Shu KH, Cheng CH, et al. Long-term impact of hepatitis B, C virus infection on renal transplantation. *Am J Nephrol.* 2001;21:300-306.

8. Bruchfeld A, Wilczek H, Elinder CG. Hepatitis C infection, time in renal-replacement therapy, and outcome after kidney transplantation. *Transplantation.* 2004;78:745-750.

9. Hestin D, Guillemin F, Castin N, et al. Pretransplant hepatitis C virus infection: a predictor of proteinuria after renal transplantation. *Transplantation.* 1998;65:741-744.

10. Morales JM. Hepatitis C virus infection and renal disease after renal transplantation. *Transplant Proc.* 2004;36:760-762.

11. Ozdemir BH, Ozdemir FN, Sezer S, et al. De novo glomerulonephritis in renal allografts with hepatitis C virus infection. *Transplant Proc.* 2006;38:492-495.

12. Cruzado JM, Casanovas-Taltavull T, Torras J, et al. Pretransplant interferon prevents hepatitis C virus-associated glomerulonephritis in renal allografts by HCV-RNA clearance. *Am J Transplant.* 2003;3:357-360.

13. Cruzado JM, Carrera M, Torras J, et al. Hepatitis C virus infection and de novo glomerular lesions in renal allografts. *Am J Transplant.* 2001;1:171-178.

14. Gürsoy M, Güvener N, Köksal R, et al. Impact of HCV infection on development of post-transplantation diabetes mellitus in renal allograft recipients. *Transplant Proc.* 2000;32:561-562.

15. Fabrizi F, Martin P, Dixit V, et al. Post-transplant diabetes mellitus and HCV seropositive status after renal transplantation: meta-analysis of clinical studies. *Am J Transplant.* 2005;5:2433-2440.

16. Hjelmesaeth J, Harmann A, Leivestad T, et al. The impact of early-diagnosed new-onset post-transplant ion diabetes mellitus on survival and major cardiovascular events. *Kidney Int.* 2006;69:588-595.

17. Fabrizi F, Dixit V, Messa P, et al. Interferon monotherapy of chronic hepatitis C in dialysis patients: meta-analysis of clinical trials. *J Viral Hepat.* 2008;15:79-88.

18. Fabrizi F, Dixit V, Messa P, et al. Pegylated interferon monotherapy of chronic hepatitis C in dialysis patients: meta-analysis of clinical trials. *J Med Virol.* 2010;82:768-775.

19. Barril G, Quiroga JA, Sanz P, et al. Pegylated interferon-alpha2a kinetics during experimental hemodialysis: impact of permeability and pore size of dialysers. *Aliment Pharmacol Ther.* 2004;20:37-44.

20. Bruchfeld A, Stahle L, Andersson J, et al. Ribavirin treatment in dialysis patients with chronic hepatitis C virus infection—a pilot study. *J Viral Hepatol.* 2001;8:287-292.

21. Mousa DH, Abdalla AH, Al-Shoail G, et al. Alpha-interferon with ribavirin in the treatment of hemodialysis patients with hepatitis C. *Transplant Proc.* 2004;36:1831-1834.

22. van Leusen R, Adang RP, de Vries RA, et al. Pegylated interferon alfa-2a (40kD) and ribavirin in haemodialysis patients with chronic hepatitis C. *Nephrol Dial Transplant.* 2008;23:721-725.

23. Rendina M, Schena A, Castellaneta NM, et al. The treatment of chronic hepatitis C with peginterferon alfa-2a (40kDa) plus ribavirin in haemodialysed patients awaiting renal transplant. *J Hepatol.* 2007;46:768-774.

24. Fissell RB, Bragg-Gresham JL, Woods JD, et al. Patterns of hepatitis C prevalence and seroconversion in hemodialysis units from three continents: the DOPPS. *Kidney Int.* 2004;65:2335-2342.

25. Berenguer M. Treatment of chronic hepatitis C in hemodialysis patients. *Hepatology.* 2008;48:1690-1699.

26. Fabrizi F, Martin P, Dixit V, et al. Meta-analysis: effect of hepatitis C virus on mortality in dialysis. *Aliment Pharmacol Ther.* 2004;20:1271-1277.

27. Fabrizi F, Takkouche B, Lunghi G, et al. The impact of hepatitis C virus infection on survival in dialysis patients: meta-analysis of observational studies. *J Viral Hepat.* 2007;14:697-703.

28. Di Napoli A, Pezzotti P, Di Lallo D, et al. Epidemiology of hepatitis C virus among long-term dialysis patients: a 9-year study in an Italian region. *Am J Kidney Disease.* 2006;48:629-637.

29. Kalantar-Zadeh K, McAllister CJ, Miller LG. Clinical characteristics and mortality in hepatitis C-positive haemodialysis patients: a population based study. *Nephrol Dial Transplant.* 2005;20:1662-1669.

30. Fried MW. Side effects of therapy of hepatitis C and their management. *Hepatology.* 2002;36:S237-S244.

31. Russo MW, Fried MW. Side effects of therapy for chronic hepatitis C. *Gastroenterology.* 2003;124:1711-1719.

32. Fabrizi F, Martin P. Management of HCV in dialysis patients. In: Foster GB, Reddy KR, eds. *Clinical Dilemmas in Viral Liver Disease.* 1st ed. Hoboken, NJ: Wiley-Blackwell; 2010:50-54.

33. Kramer TH, Gaar GG, Ray CG, et al. Hemodialysis clearance of intravenously administered ribavirin. *Antimicrob Agents Chemother.* 1990;34:489-490.

34. Kalia H, Lopez PM, Martin P. Treatment of HCV in patients with renal failure. *Arch Med Res.* 2007;38:628-633.

35. Fabrizi F, Dulai G, Dixit V, et al. Meta-analysis: interferon for the treatment of chronic hepatitis C in dialysis patients. *Aliment Pharmacol Ther.* 2003;18:1071-1081.

36. Covic A, Maftei ID, Mardare NG, et al. Analysis of safety and efficacy of pegylated interferon alpha-2a in hepatitis C virus positive hemodialysis patients: results from a large multicenter audit. *J Nephrol.* 2006;19:794-801.

37. Tan SS, Abu Hassan MR, Abdullah A, et al. Safety and efficacy of an escalating dose regimen of pegylated interferon alpha-2b in the treatment of haemodialysis patients with chronic hepatitis C. *J Viral Hepatol.* 2010;17:410-418.

38. Bruchfeld A, Lindahl K, Reichard O, et al. Pegylated interferon and ribavirin treatment for hepatitis C in haemodialysis patients. *J Viral Hepat.* 2006;13:316-321.

39. Carriero D, Fabrizi F, Uriel AJ, et al. Treatment of dialysis patients with chronic hepatitis C using pegylated interferon and low-dose ribavirin. *Int J Artif Organs.* 2008;31:295-302.

40. Fuller TC, Delmonico FL, Cosimi B, et al. The impact of blood transfusion on renal transplantation. *Ann Surg.* 1978;187:211-218.

41. Sezer S, Ozdemir FN, Akcay A, et al. Renal transplantation offers a better survival in HCV-infected ESRD patients. *Clin Transplant.* 2004;18:619-623.

42. Okoh EJ, Bucci JR, Simon JF, et al. HCV in patients with end-stage renal disease. *Am J Gastroenterol.* 2008;103:2123-2134.

RETRANSPLANTATION FOR SEVERE RECURRENT HEPATITIS C VIRUS AND PREVIOUSLY FAILED PEGYLATED-INTERFERON/ RIBAVIRIN THERAPY

Vandana Khungar, MD, MSc; Tyralee Goo, MD; and Fred Poordad, MD

Hepatitis C is the leading indication for liver transplantation in the United States and Europe. Recurrence in the graft is almost universal and often leads to graft dysfunction or failure. Treatment with interferon-based therapies, to date, have yielded poor results, and many patients require retransplantation. Given the shortage of liver grafts, offering a second transplant to an individual while many are still waiting for their first is a difficult decision, particularly if the outcomes are poor.

In this section, a debate based on available literature assesses whether or not it is feasible and cost effective to retransplant recurrent hepatitis C. As with many controversies, the data is not always clear or understood, and progress in medical science may ultimately change the argument.

Jensen D.
*Controversies in Hepatology: The Experts Analyze Both
Sides (pp 61-72)*
© 2011 SLACK Incorporated

POINT

Patients With Recurrent Hepatitis C Virus and Previously Failed Pegylated-Interferon/Ribavirin Therapy Should Be Retransplanted

by Vandana Khungar, MD, MSc

Hepatitis C virus (HCV) infection is the leading cause for orthotopic liver transplantation (OLT) in the United States and Europe. HCV infection occurs almost universally after liver transplantation (90% after 5 years)[1] and fibrosis progression and clinical decompensation occur at an accelerated rate in the new graft.[2] The median interval from infection to cirrhosis is 9.5 years in OLT recipients compared to 30 years in immunocompetent patients.[3] It is not clear that rapid fibrosis progression in the first graft will recur at the same rate in the second graft. After antiviral treatment with pegylated-interferon (PEG) and ribavirin (RBV) fail, retransplantation (RT) is the only option to achieve long-term survival in the patient who develops decompensated cirrhosis from recurrent HCV. As with other controversies in organ transplantation, the issues of resource utilization, cost-benefit ratios, and ethics must be addressed for RT in recurrent HCV. When appropriate patients are chosen using prognostic scores and the timing of transplant is optimized, it is clear that patients with recurrent HCV and previously failed PEG/RBV should be retransplanted. The lack of prospective data and initially discouraging results may hinder patients with HCV from receiving RT, but all data must be interpreted with caution and decisions made on a case-by-case basis. Several randomized, controlled trials have been conducted to address this question and are detailed in Table 7-1.

Survival Rates Not as Low as They Initially Appeared

RT for all indications is associated with longer hospital stays, greater cost, and decreased survival.[4,5] It initially appeared that outcomes in RT for HCV were worse than for other indications. The Scientific Registry of Transplant Recipients database cohort of 1700 patients included 500 with HCV. A retrospective analysis of this cohort found a 31% higher covariate-adjusted mortality risk in HCV-infected recipients compared to all other recipients combined.[6] A caveat to this data is that there was a large amount of heterogeneity in the non-HCV-infected group and there was a lack of data on the specific indications for RT in this analysis. Two studies, one from Europe and one from UCLA, demonstrated no overall difference in outcomes of RT in patients with and without HCV.[5,7] The only groups found to have better outcomes are patients with hepatitis B and autoimmune hepatitis. Those patients with cryptogenic cirrhosis and alcohol-related disease have similar outcomes to HCV patients.[8,9]

When indicators of severity are controlled for, HCV may not independently predict poor outcomes.[10,11] Data from 10 centers shows no difference in 1- and 3-year survival rates in HCV and non-HCV patients.[12] This same study revealed that one-third of patients with HCV-related graft failure are not considered candidates for RT and only half of those who are evaluated are listed. Ghabrial et al[13] demonstrated that in 1034 HCV-infected patients and 1249 non-HCV-infected patients who underwent OLT between 1994 and 2005, patient and graft survival were significantly lower for HCV-infected compared to non-HCV-infected patients who underwent RT at least 90 days after primary OLT. On multivariate analysis, the

Table 7-1.

Randomized Controlled Trials of Antiviral Treatment in Recurrent HCV

AUTHOR	Gane[27] 1998	Cotter[28] 2001	Chalasani[29] 2005	Carrion[30] 2007	Angelico[31] 2007
PATIENT POPULATION	Recurrent HCV	Noncirrhotic recurrent HCV	Noncirrhotic recurrent HCV without cholestatic fibrosing hepatitis	Mild recurrent HCV (fibrosis stage F0 – F2) Severe recurrent HCV* (F3, F4, cholestatic hepatitis)	Noncirrhotic OLT with recurrent HCV
NUMBER OF PATIENTS	A: 14 B: 14 Total 28	A: 4 B: 8 Total 12	A: 32 B: 33 Total 67	A: 27 B: 27 C: 27* Total 81	A: 21 B: 21 Total 42
REGIMEN	A: IFN- α [3 mU TIW] B: Ribavirin [1-1.2 g/d weight based x 24 wks	A: Control B: IFN [3 mU/d x 12 months]	A: Control B: PEG(α-2a) [180 µg/wk x 48 wks]	A: Control B: PEG/RBV C: PEG/RBV * [PEG 1.5 µg/kg/wk x 48 wks] [RBV 800 to 1200 mg/d based on CrCl]	A:PEG/RBV B:PEG [PEG:180 µg /wk x 48 wks] [RBV 200 mg/d, increased 100 mg every 15 d to max tolerated]
SVR	A: 0% B: 0%	A: 0% B: 12.5%	A: 0 % B: 12%	A: 0% B: 48% C: 18.5%*	A: 33% B: 38%
CONCLUSION	No SVR achieved with monotherapy of IFN or RBV.	Low daily doses IFN (α-2a) provided histological benefit.	PEG is safe and tolerable with some efficacy in post-LT patients. Treatment group had significantly lower fibrosis scores at 48 wks but not at 72 wks suggesting short-term histological benefit.	Antiviral tx slows disease progression in SVR responders. SVR achieved in 16% of genotype 1 and 34% of non-genotype 1 patients.	No difference in SVR due to inability to sustain full doses of anti-virals and lack of Ribavirin booster effect. Both regimens associated with adverse events including acute rejection and need for dose reductions. EVR associated with 50% chance of SVR.

(continued)

Table 7-1 (continued).

RANDOMIZED CONTROLLED TRIALS OF ANTIVIRAL TREATMENT IN RECURRENT HCV

AUTHOR	Samuel[32] 2003	Nair[33] 2008	Lodato[34] 2008	Gordon[35] 2005	Ghalib[36] 2006
PATIENT POPULATION	Recurrent HCV >6 months after transplant, Metavir score >1	Recurrent HCV	Genotype 1 recurrent HCV Previous nonresponders to IFN + RBV included.	Recurrent HCV	Recurrent HCV
NUMBER OF PATIENTS	A: 28 B: 24 Total 52	A: 13 B: 17 Total 30	A: 23 B: 9 C: 9 Total 41	A: 9 B: 4 Total 13	A: 32 B: 27 Total 59
REGIMEN	A: IFN + RBV [IFN 3 mU TIW + RBV 400-600 mg BID x 48 wks] B: No treatment	A: Amantadine + PEG/RBV [Amantadine 200 mg/d + PEG 1 µg/kg/wk + RBV 800 mg/d x 52 weeks] B: PEG-IFN +RBV [PEG 1 µg/kg/wk + RBV 800 mg/d x 52 weeks]	A, B, and C: PEG + RBV [PEG 1 µg/kg/wk + RBV 8-10 mg/kg/d x 24 wks] A: If EVR, PEG+RBV x 24 more weeks B: No EVR, PEG + RBV x 24 more weeks C: No EVR, stop treatment	A: PEG + RBV [PEG 1.5 µg/kg/wk + RBV 200 mg BID then 400 mg BID x 52 wks] B: PEG + RBV [PEG 0.5 µg/kg/wk + RBV 200 mg BID then 400 mg BID x 52 wks]	A: PEG+RBV [PEG 0.5 µg/d x 4 wks then 1.5 µg/d x 48 wks + RBV 600 mg/d then 800 mg/d at 4 wks] B: PEG+RBV [PEG 0.5 µg/d x 52 wks + RBV 600 mg/d then 800 mg/d at 4 wks]
SVR	A: 21.4% B: 0%	A: 26% B: 50%	A: 48% B: 11% C: 0%	A: 77.8% B: 50%	A: 59.4% B: 18.5%
CONCLUSION	SVR in 21% of transplant recipients but many discontinued therapy due to side effects. Lower doses of ribavirin need to be studied.	The data is encouraging for 1 year of treatment using a steroid free regimen.	PEG-IFN alfa-2b is effective in one out of 4 patients with HCV genotype 1 after LT. Treatment should be discontinued in patients with no virological response at week 12.	SVR was achieved in 69.2%. PEG dose did not determine SVR EPO may improve SVR by allowing continued full dose therapy. SVR did not confer improved histology in all patients.	SVR is higher in those on high dose PEG (α-2b) and non-genotype 1 patients (68.8% versus 30.2% in genotype 1).

only independent predictors of mortality were recipient age, MELD >25, RT during the first year after OLT, donor age >60, and a warm ischemia time >75 minutes. The International Liver Transplantation Society Expert Panel[14] determined that bilirubin >10 mg/dL, creatinine >2.0 mg/dL, recipient age >55, donor age >40, and early HCV recurrence (cirrhosis <1 year after OLT) were associated with worse outcome after RT. The poor outcome in patients with early HCV recurrence may be due to poor liver function in those with cholestatic hepatitis C at the time of RT. The time between first and second transplants is a strong predictor of success, with the highest death rate in one series being 8 to 30 days after first transplant. This variable is not routinely adjusted for in studies looking at RT for HCV.[15]

Prognostic Scores Should Be Used as Tools to Determine Candidacy for Retransplantation

As more is learned about risk factors for poor outcomes, models based on logistic regression analysis of donor and recipient variables have been developed to assist in decision making for patients listed for RT. There are models for urgent (primary nonfunction or hepatic artery thrombosis) and elective indications for RT. Recurrent HCV with failed PEG/RBV is an elective indication for RT. Scores appropriate for this setting include the Rosen score,[16] the MELD score,[8,13,17] the Child-Pugh score,[17-19] and the Donor Risk Index (DRI). Variables with the highest impact on survival are the serum bilirubin and creatinine. The Rosen (R) score is based on a study that analyzed recipient age, bilirubin, creatinine, and retransplant interval time in 773 patients who underwent RT. Patients with an R score ≤16 had the best 1- and 3-year survival of 75% and 70%, while survival for those with R scores ≥20.5 was 42% and 38%, respectively. The Rosen score was highly predictive of survival but has not been rigorously validated. One study evaluated the MELD score in 2129 retransplant candidates from 1996 to 2002.[8] Survival after RT did not differ for HCV-infected patients in comparison with other causes of elective RT (metabolic, genetic, alcohol, cryptogenic, primary biliary cirrhosis, primary sclerosing cholangitis), and only autoimmune hepatitis and hepatitis B showed a higher survival. A MELD score >25 was a risk factor for lower short-term survival after RT.

Bussutil[15] and Ghobrial[11] developed a model to calculate survival based on recipient and donor age, creatinine, bilirubin, prothrombin time, and warm and cold ischemia times. The same authors substituted the preoperative serum creatinine, bilirubin, and prothrombin values for the MELD score and included the time between first and second transplantation. They reported a 1-year survival benefit >65% in 30- to 40-year-old recipients with any MELD score and in 50-year-old candidates with a MELD <24. From these data, the authors recommended avoiding RT in older recipients or those with a MELD >28.[11] This score was validated using the UNOS database with excellent accuracy. The DRI developed by Feng et al[20] uses 7 donor variables that independently predicted a higher risk of graft failure after RT: donor age >40 years (particularly >60 years), donation after cardiac death, split/partial grafts, African-American race, low height, cerebrovascular accident, and time to transplantation.

RT should be used judiciously in patients with a reasonable survival probability as indicated by well-validated prognostic scores. Determining at what predicted survival rate the procedure is unacceptable is an important development, as prediction models are ineffective when the survival rate they predict cannot be used in clinical decision making.[21] These scores have shown an improvement in survival in HCV-infected patients after RT, approaching similar rates as those obtained in non-HCV-infected patients. Several models demonstrated a group of patients with a high risk of death after RT: candidates with a Markmann score >2.3,[22] Rosen score ≥20.5,[16] Child-Pugh score ≥10,[17] MELD >25,[8] or Linhares model >36.[23] RT in these patients should be avoided (Table 7-2).

Table 7-2.	
PREDICTIVE MODELS TO DETERMINE CANDIDACY FOR RETRANSPLANTATION	
Rosen Score	Recipient age, bilirubin, creatinine, interval to re-OLT
MELD	Creatinine, bilirubin, INR, dialysis status
Child-Turcotte-Pugh	Bilirubin, albumin, INR, ascites, encephalopathy
Donor Risk Index (DRI)	Age, donation after cardiac death, split/partial grafts, race, height, cause of death, organ location (local, regional, national), cold time
Markmann	Cold ischemia time, ventilator status, preoperative creatinine, preoperative bilirubin, age group (child or adult)
Linhares	Recipient age, creatinine, urgency of retransplantation, early failure of the first graft
Busuttil and Ghobrial	Recipient age, recipient creatinine, donor gender, urgent UNOS status, donor age, bilirubin, prothrombin time, retransplantation, warm and cold ischemia times

Hepatitis C Treatment Is Evolving

Not only are the survival rates in patients with recurrent HCV and previously failed PEG/RBV underestimated and patients sometimes inappropriately selected, but patients will soon have better antiviral regiments to treat recurrent hepatitis C in their grafts. After HCV patients undergo transplant, it is currently very difficult to balance immune suppression or treatment of rejection in the setting of recurrent hepatitis C. The new generation of protease inhibitors may assist in this optimal regimen. With new therapies, patients should be treated while on the waitlist to suppress viral loads and increase survival while awaiting RT. The International Liver Transplantation Society Expert Panel[14] established guidelines for the administration of antiviral treatment if moderate to severe (grade 3 or 4) inflammation or significant fibrosis (stage 2) was present in protocol liver biopsies. Currently, antiviral treatment with PEG/RBV has low SVR rates of approximately 30% to 40% according to 2 systematic reviews.[24,25] Even in those who have biochemical response but do not achieve SVR, stabilization and improvement in liver fibrosis and portal pressure in patients has been described.[26] It remains to be seen if the protease inhibitors will be effective in treating post-transplant patients who previously failed PEG/RBV, but results for pre-transplant failures of PEG/RBV have been encouraging.[37]

Summary

Careful examination of the literature reveals that certain patient populations are better suited for RT for recurrent HCV after PEG/RBV failure. One cannot make a blanket statement that RT should be avoided for all patients with recurrent HCV. Rather, appropriate patient selection through the use of well-validated prognostic scores can improve survival. The best way to prevent RT in HCV-infected patients is to administer early antiviral treatment to patients with fibrosis, moderate or severe inflammation, or portal hypertension soon after initial transplant, as these patients are at high risk of severe hepatitis C recurrence. As current antiviral therapy only eradicates HCV infection in 30% to 40% of patients, RT may be inevitable for individuals progressing to graft cirrhosis. With newer hepatitis C therapies, initial and retransplanted graft survival will likely be increased. RT of patients with severe recurrent HCV and previously failed PEG/RBV therapy is a necessity due to the universal reinfection in transplanted grafts.

KEY POINTS

■ HCV is the leading cause for OLT in the United States and Europe and reinfection occurs almost universally after transplant.

■ Retransplantation is the only way to achieve long-term survival in patients with recurrent HCV.

■ Survival data for patients who received RT for HCV are higher than initially thought.

■ When validated prognostic scores are used to determine candidacy for RT, this further increases survival rates.

■ Newer medications for HCV will further increase graft survival and may be an option to treat patients who previously failed PEG/RBV and have undergone RT.

COUNTERPOINT

Patients With Recurrent Hepatitis C Virus Who Previously Failed Pegylated-Interferon/ Ribavirin Therapy Should Not Be Treated With Retransplantation

by Tyralee Goo, MD

Chronic hepatitis C infection affects an estimated 180 million people worldwide. In the United States and Europe, hepatitis C is the most common indication (40%) for OLT.[8,26] Recurrence of HCV infection after liver transplantation is a universal occurrence in patients with detectable viral load at time of transplant. The natural history of recurrent HCV is an accelerated course to liver fibrosis, cirrhosis, and decompensation. Histologic evidence of acute hepatitis C is seen between 4 to 12 weeks after transplantation with progression to chronic hepatitis in 70% to 90% at 1 year.[38] Cirrhosis occurs in recurrent HCV with a median time of 10 years compared to 30 years in the immune-competent chronic HCV population.[39] In addition, hepatic decompensation after cirrhosis at 1 year (>40% as compared to <5%) and survival at 3 years (<10% as compared to >60%)[2,40] are remarkably different in the recurrent HCV and chronic HCV patients, respectively. When standard therapy of PEG/RBV is not an option due to nonresponse or clinical decompensation, recurrent HCV cases are considered for retransplantation. Patients that fail PEG/RBV are unlikely to attain sustained viral clearance with any other current regimens. After retransplantation, the HCV recurs in the majority and leads to graft damage again. Additionally, there is a high rate of mortality seen after retransplantation that is related to advanced disease state present at the time of retransplantation. Donor livers are a scarce resource for which scrutinizing decisions must be made to optimize allocation. Given the scarceness of this resource, it is critical to strive for successful transplant outcomes. In consideration of this, recurrent HCV patients with prior failure of PEG/IFN should not be candidates for RT.

Resource Allocation: Retransplantation Is Associated With Increased Costs and Decreased Survival Rates

The United Network of Organ Sharing (UNOS) OPTN database listed 6101 deceased donor liver transplantations that occurred in 2009 of which 453 (7%) were RT patients. There are approximately 16,000 people (as of September 2010) in the United States on the waiting list for a liver transplant.[41] As the demand for donor livers outweighs the supply available greater than 2:1, careful consideration must be taken to ensure judicial allocation and maximum utility. The costs of liver RT are composed of both the inherent value of the limited graft supply and the financial health care costs. On average, liver transplantation costs between $414,000 to $738,000 and increases with disease severity as measured by the MELD score.[42] RT costs are up to 40% higher than primary transplant,[43] and a multicenter US study showed that length of stay in the hospital was about 1 week longer than primary transplantation hospitalization.[44]

Retransplantation outcomes with regard to patient and graft survival demonstrates overall poorer outcomes. In chronic hepatitis C, patient survival rate is significantly different at 1, 3, and 5 years for primary versus retransplanted subjects (86%, 76%, 68% versus 61%, 50%, 45%, respectively), as demonstrated in UNOS data from 1996 to 2002.[8] Retrospective data reveal chronic hepatitis C patients have decreased survival after RT compared to hepatitis B and autoimmune hepatitis patients. However, there is no significant difference compared with other non-HCV liver disease indications.[8,44] Five-year survival is significantly decreased to less than 60% in all patients with MELD >25 and recurrent HCV patients with MELD >20 at time of RT.[8] A multicenter study found 3-year survival in HCV-infected patients after RT regardless of MELD score was 40% to 56%.[44] Specific groups of severe recurrent HCV patients who have particularly dismal outcomes with RT include those with fibrosing cholestatic disease, early HCV recurrence, and renal dysfunction.[44] While recurrent HCV alone is not associated with poorer outcomes after retransplantation, there is a high risk for mortality associated with RT in general and it is significantly higher than in primary transplant mortality. Additionally, the current use of MELD scoring in selection of graft candidates will tend to prioritize the clinically sicker patient who is likely weaker and shown to have worse survival outcomes after the second graft. RT is a higher risk surgery with increased morbidity and mortality. Liver RT in the United States has decreased over time, composing 23% of OLT in 1990, 10% in 2000, and 7% in 2009.[41] This may be the result of many institutions becoming reluctant to perform these procedures for HCV patients,[44] allowing graft resources to be directed toward primary transplants or well-compensated retransplants for non-HCV recurrence.

Retreatment and New Therapies Offer Some Promise for Nonresponders

Failure of therapy with standard of care PEG/RBV is a problem that affects up to 60% of genotype 1 and 30% of genotype 2 and 3 patients. The efficacy of retreatment in prior PEG/RBV nonresponders has been examined in the pre-liver transplant population.[45-47] The REPEAT trial achieved up to 16% SVR using RBV and high-dose PEG for an extended treatment course in a predominantly genotype 1 population.[45] In advanced fibrosis, using an extended course of PEG/RBV has demonstrated an SVR of approximately 6%.[46] Higher success rates correlated with genotype 2 and 3, lower baseline viral loads, and less advanced fibrosis.[46] Synthetic consensus interferon is another treatment option studied in chronic HCV PEG/RBV nonresponders with SVR reported from 6.9%[47] to 37%[48] in a predominantly genotype 1 population; however, predictably only 4.5%[47] SVR is seen in patients with cirrhosis. While the Cochrane systematic review of antiviral therapy in recurrent HCV reported no difference in the primary outcomes of mortality, graft rejection, or RT,[49] other studies have shown that in recurrent HCV, achieving

SVR reduces mortality[50] and antiviral treatment can decrease graft fibrosis progression[28-30] and improve hemodynamics.[30] Despite the modest SVR rates achieved in retreatment of chronic HCV nonresponders, similar outcomes may be attainable in select recurrent HCV patients. Unfortunately, no randomized controlled study in the recurrent HCV population post-transplantation has yet to examine the efficacy of retreatment in PEG/RBV nonresponders. Considering the beneficial effects of antiviral therapy on graft preservation, it is prudent to explore this option in recurrent HCV.

The incoming era of direct antiviral therapies offer tremendous hope for prior nonresponders. The protease inhibitor class of drugs utilized in triple combination therapy with Peg-IFN and RBV studied in genotype 1 nonresponders has demonstrated up to 39% SVR.[51] While these studies did not include transplanted subjects, it is reasonable to expect some success achieving SVR using these medical therapy options after OLT. Poorer outcomes would be expected with more advanced graft fibrosis, and possibly poorer medication tolerance. However, in consideration of the shortage of grafts available and inevitable HCV recurrence after retransplantation, it is a fair argument to try to stem the need for RT through retreatment regimens using direct-acting antiviral therapies.

Summary

Currently, there are no nationwide guidelines to direct clinical decision making regarding liver RT. Retrospective data have more recently established that RT outcomes do not significantly differ between HCV and non-HCV patients. However, poorer outcomes occur with RT compared with primary transplants. Single-center studies of RT for recurrent HCV report 3-year patient survival rates between 33% and 76%.[52-54] The significant differential is likely due to center-specific variances of patient demographics, clinical experience, as well as factors at time of RT associated with poorer outcomes such as advanced donor age >60 years,[52] MELD >25,[8] cirrhosis,[52] elevated creatinine, bilirubin, prolonged ischemia times, and others. These factors, seen as predictive tools for RT outcome, have been formulated into prognostication scoring systems to identify high-risk candidates in whom RT would not be reasonable. The Markmann,[7] Rosen,[16] MELD, Child-Pugh, and DRI are all scoring models that have been used to help achieve ethical allocation and improve successful outcomes in RT.[37] There has been no comparison study between the different prognostic models, and at this time no consensus exists regarding the most effective model or the minimal acceptable outcome of survival. All measures should be taken to slow fibrosis progression in these patients as tolerated, including retreatment regimens, new therapies, diabetes control,[55] and avoidance of advanced age donor grafts and high-dose corticosteroids.[37] However, until a validated prognostication model can be uniformly implemented to ensure a judicious assignment of liver grafts with reproducible survival outcomes, it is a reasonable decision not to pursue RT in severe recurrent patients, particularly those who have previously failed therapy.

KEY POINTS

- Chronic HCV will recur in retransplanted graft if viral clearance is not achieved.
- Donor livers are a scarce resource with demand outnumbering supply >2:1.
- Retransplantation is associated with elevated health care cost, longer hospitalization, and with greater morbidity and mortality over primary OLT.
- Decreased graft fibrosis can be achieved with SVR.
- Studies show some efficacy with using antivirals and new protease inhibitors on prior nonresponders, which may be promising for the post-transplant population; however, studies need to be performed.
- There are currently no national guidelines regarding selection of RT candidates, a validated prognostication scoring system, or uniformly accepted outcome measures.

EXPERT OPINION

Retransplantation of Recurrent Hepatitis C: There Is No Right Answer

by Fred Poordad, MD

Hepatitis C recurrence after transplantation is one of the more challenging clinical scenarios in transplantation medicine. While there are some predictive factors that portend a poor outcome in this population, the organ shortage precludes an overly selective process for graft selection for the hepatitis C patient. Over the past 20 years, as organ recipients have been allocated organs at a later stage of their disease, it has likely affected the outcomes and perhaps the need for RT. Excessive immune suppression may have negative implications on outcomes, but it has been hard to determine if specific immune-suppression regimens affect recurrence rates or histologic severity. Hence, there is apparently little that can be done to alter recurrence post-transplantation with either pre-transplant selection or post-transplant immune modulation. Recurrence does occur and the severity of it appears largely unpredictable.

Antiviral treatment of recurrent disease is certainly warranted, although outcomes are not assured and most studies have shown poor sustained response rates, particularly in genotype 1 patients. Those who clear virus appear to do well, however, and with evolving direct-acting antiviral therapies, response rates will undoubtedly improve. Indeed, this may allow for greater clearance rates of virus before and after transplantation, altering the natural history of disease.

When treatment fails after transplantation, the only known viable alternative therapy is RT. This option has led to some success, but also many failures with re-recurrence of severe HCV and failure of the second graft. It is very difficult to make a sweeping generalization whether or not to repeat transplantation for failed grafts in the HCV patient, particularly since the overall outcomes are not drastically different from RT for other conditions. However, there are clearly some subsets of patients that need further assessment to determine if RT is truly futile, such as those with very rapid recurrence or cholestatic features, significant muscle wasting, and renal failure. However, even in this population, if the original organ was suboptimal or if there were perioperative complications, it is difficult to deny RT.

There is little to support a rigid stance either in support of or against RT. Like many things in the medical field, there is a lack of concrete data and consensus on how to approach this patient population. Additionally, as therapies evolve and increased clearance rates are realized, outcomes may very well change and a consensus may develop over time. Until then, it is reasonable and prudent to selectively retransplant patients using good clinical judgment. Direct-acting antiviral therapy will need to be assessed in this population to determine if outcomes can be affected, and thereby bring clarity to what the optimal treatment should be for post-transplant HCV patient.

References

1. Berenguer M. Natural history of recurrent hepatitis C. *Liver Transpl.* 2002;8(10Suppl1):S14-S18.
2. Berenguer M, Prieto M, Rayon JM, et al. Natural history of clinically compensated hepatitis C virus-related graft cirrhosis after liver tranplantation. *Hepatology.* 2000;32(4Pt1):852-858.
3. Prieto M, Berenguer M, Rayon JM, et al. High incidence of allograft cirrhosis in hepatitis C virus genotype 1b infection following transplantation: relationship with rejection episodes. *Hepatology.* 1999;29(1):250-256.
4. Biggins SW, Terrault NA. Should HCV-related cirrhosis be a contraindication for retranpslantation? *Liver Transpl.* 2003;9(3):236-238.
5. Azoulay D, Linhares MM, Huguet E, et al. Decision for retransplantation of the liver: an experience- and cost-based analysis. *Ann Surg.* 2002;236(6):713-721.
6. Pelletier SJ, Schaubel DE, Punch JD, et al. Hepatitis C is a risk factor for death after liver retransplantation. *Liver Transpl.* 2005;11(4):434-440.
7. Markmann JF, Markowitz JS, Yersiz H, et al. Long-term survival after retransplantation of the liver. *Ann Surg.* 1997;226(4):408-418.
8. Watt KDS, Lyden ER, McCashland TM. Poor survivial after liver retransplantation: is hepatitis C to blame? *Liver Transpl.* 2003;9:1019-1024.
9. McCashland TM. Retransplantation for recurrent hepatitis C: positive aspects. *Liver Transpl.* 2003;9(11): S67-S72.
10. Rosen HR, Madden JP, Martin P. A model to predict survival following liver retransplantation. *Hepatology.* 1999;29(2):365-370.
11. Ghobrial RM, Gornbein J, Steadman R, et al. Pretransplant model to predict posttransplant survival in liver transplant patients. *Ann Surg.* 2002;236(3):315-322.
12. McCashland T, Watt K, Lyden E, et al. Retransplantation for hepatitis C: results of a U.S. multicenter retransplant study. *Liver Transpl.* 2007;13(9):1246-1253.
13. Ghabril M, Dickson R, Wiesner R. Improving outcomes of liver retransplantation: an analysis of trends and impact of hepatitis C infection. *Am J Transplant.* 2008;8(2):404-411.
14. Wiesner RH, Sorrell M, Villamil F, et al. Report of the first International Liver Transplantation Society expert panel consensus conference on liver transplantation and hepatitis C. *Liver Transpl.* 2003;9(11):S1-S9.
15. Busuttil RW, Farmer DG, Yersiz H, et al. Analysis of long-term outcomes of 3200 liver transplantations over two decades: a single-center experience. *Ann Surg.* 2005;241(6):905-916.
16. Rosen HR, Prieto M, Casanovas-Taltavull T, et al. Validation and refinement of survival models for liver retransplantation. *Hepatology.* 2003;38(2):460-469.
17. Yao FY, Saab S, Bass NM, et al. Prediction of survival after liver retransplantation for late graft failure based on preoperative prognostic scores. *Hepatology.* 2004;39(1):230-238.
18. Neff GW, O'Brien CB, Nery J, et al. Factors that identify survival after liver retransplantation for allograft failure caused by recurrent hepatitis C infection. *Liver Transpl.* 2004;10(12):1497-1503.
19. Marti J, Charco R, Ferrer J, et al. Optimization of liver grafts in liver retransplantation: a European single-center experience. *Surgery.* 2008;144(5):762-769.
20. Feng S, Goodrich NP, Bragg-Gresham JL, et al. Characteristics associated with liver graft failure: the concept of a donor risk index. *Am J Transplant.* 2006;6(4):783-790.
21. Verna EC, Brown RS Jr. Hepatitis C and liver transplantation: enhancing outcomes and should patients be retransplanted. *Clin Liver Dis.* 2008;12(3):637-659.
22. Markmann JF, Gornbein J, Markowitz JS, et al. A simple model to estimate survival after retransplantation of the liver. *Transplantation.* 1999;67(3):422-430.
23. Linhares MM, Azoulay D, Matos D, et al. Liver retransplantation: a model for determining long-term survival. *Transplantation.* 2006;81(7):1016-1021.
24. Berenguer M. Systematic review of the treatment of established recurrent hepatitis C with pegylated interferon in combination with ribavirin. *J Hepatol.* 2008;49(2):274-287.
25. Xirouchakis E, Triantos C, Manousou P, et al. Pegylated-interferon and ribavirin in liver transplant candidates and recipients with HCV cirrhosis: systematic review and meta-analysis of prospective controlled studies. *J Viral Hepat.* 2008;15(10):699-709.

26. Brown RS. Hepatitis C and liver transplantation. *Nature*. 2005;436(7053):973-978.
27. Gane EJ, Lo SK, Riordan SM, et al. A randomized study comparing ribavirin and interferon alfa mono-therapy for hepatitis C recurrence after liver transplantation. *Hepatology*. 1998;27(5):1403-1407.
28. Cotler SJ, Ganger DR, Kaur S, et al. Daily interferon therapy for hepatitis C virus infection in liver transplant recipients. *Transplantation*. 2001;71(2):261-266.
29. Chalasani N, Manzarbeitia C, Ferenci P, et al. Peginterferon alfa-2a for hepatitis C after liver transplanta-tion: two randomized, controlled trials. *Hepatology*. 2005;41(2):289-298.
30. Carrion JA, Navasa M, Garcia-Retortillo M, et al. Efficacy of antiviral therapy on hepatitis C recurrence after liver transplantation: a randomized controlled study. *Gastroenterology*. 2007;132:1746-1756.
31. Angelico M, Petrolati A, Lionetti R, et al. A randomized study on peg-interferon alfa-2a with or without ribavirin in liver transplant recipients with recurrent hepatitis C. *J Hepatol*. 2007;46(6):1009-1017.
32. Samuel D, Bizollon T, Feray C, et al. Interferon-alpha 2b plus ribavirin in patients with chronic hepatitis C after liver transplantation: a randomized study. *Gastroenterology*. 2003;124(3):642-650.
33. Nair S, Lipscomb J, Eason J. Efficacy of interferon based antiviral therapy for recurrent hepatitis C in patients who received steroid free immunosuppression for liver transplantation. *Transplantation*. 2008;86(3):418-422.
34. Lodato F, Berardi S, Gramenzi A, et al. Clinical trial: peg-interferon alfa-2b and ribavirin for the treatment of genotype-1 hepatitis C recurrence after liver transplantation. *Alimentary Pharm Ther*. 2008;28(4):450-457.
35. Gordon FD, Morin D, Davis C, et al. High sustained virological response (SVR) in HCV treatment with peginterferon-alfa 2b (PEG) and ribavirin (RBV) after liver transplantation (LT). *Am J Transpl*. 2005;5(S11):181.
36. Ghalib R, Levine C, Hollinger B, et al. Treatment of recurrent hepatitis C after liver transplantation. *Liver Transpl*. 2006;12(5):C-29.
37. Carrion JA, Navasa M, Forns X. Retransplantation in patients with hepatitis C recurrence after liver transplantation. *J Hepatol*. 2010; doi:10.1016/j.jhep.2010.06.006.
38. Gane EJ. The natural history of recurrent hepatitis C and what influences this. *Liver Transpl*. 2008;14: S36-S44.
39. Picciotto A. Antihepatitis C virus therapy in liver transplanted patients. *Ther Clin Risk Manage*. 2006;2(1):39-44.
40. Fattovich G, Giustina G, Degos F, et al. Morbidity and mortality in compensated cirrhosis type C. *Gastroenterology*. 1997;112:463-472.
41. United Network for Organ Sharing. www.unos.org. Updated daily. Accessed September 2010.
42. Buchanan P, Dzebisashvili N, Lentine KL, et al. Liver transplantation cost in the model for end-stage liver disease era: looking beyond the transplant admission. *Liver Transpl*. 2009;15:1270-1277.
43. Evans RW, Manninen DL, Dong RB, McLynne DA. Is retransplantation cost effective? *Transplant Proc*. 1993;25:1694-1697.
44. McCashland T, Watt K, Lyden E, et al. Retransplantation for hepatitis C: results of a U.S. multicenter re-transplant study. *Liver Transpl*. 2007;13:1246-1253.
45. Jensen DM, Marcellin P, Freilich B, et al. Retreatment of patients with chronic hepatitis C who do not respond to Peginterferon-α2b. *Ann Intern Med*. 2009;150:528-540.
46. Poynard T, Colombo M, Bruix J, et al. Peginterferon alfa-2b and ribavirin: effective in patients with hepatitis C who failed interferon alfa/ribavirin therapy. *Gastroenterology*. 2009;136:1618-1628.
47. Bacon BR, Shiffman ML, Mendes F, et al. Retreating chronic hepatitis C with daily inteferon alfacon-1/ ribavirin after nonresponse to pegylated interferon/ribavirin: DIRECT results. *Hepatology*. 2009;49:1838-1846.
48. Leevy CB. Consensus interferon and ribavirin in patients with chronic hepatitis C who were nonre-sponders to pegylated interferon alfa-2b and ribavirin. *Dig Dis Sci*. 2008;53:1961-1966.
49. Gurusamy KS, Tsochatzis E, Xirouchakis E, et al. Antiviral therapy for recurrent liver graft infection with hepatitis C virus (Review). *Cochrane Database Syst Rev*. 2010;20(1):CD006803.
50. Piciotto FP, Tritto G, Lanza AG, et al. Sustained virological response to antiviral therapy reduces mortal-ity in HCV reinfection after liver transplantation. *J Hepatol*. 2007;46(3):459-465.
51. McHutchison JG, Manns MP, Muir AJ, et al. Telaprevir for previously treated chronic HCV infection. *N Engl J Med*. 2010;362:1292-1303.
52. Carmiel-Haggai M, Fiel MI, Gaddipati HC, et al. Recurrent hepatitis C after retransplantation: factors affecting graft and patient outcome. *Liver Transpl*. 2005;11(12):1567-1573.
53. Berenguer M, Prieto M, Palau A, et al. Severe recurrent hepatitis C after liver retransplantation for hepa-titis C virus-related graft cirrhosis. *Liver Transpl*. 2003;9:228-235.
54. Ghabril M, Dickson RC, Machicao VI, et al. Liver retransplantation of patients with hepatitis C infection is associated with acceptable patient and graft survival. *Liver Transpl*. 2007;13:1717-1727.
55. Veldt BJ, Poterucha JJ, Watt KD, et al. Insulin resistance, serum adipokines and risk of fibrosis progres-sion in patients transplanted for hepatitis C. *Am J Transplant*. 2009;9:1406-1413.

DOES A SUSTAINED VIROLOGIC RESPONSE AT WEEK 72 INDICATE A CURE IN CHRONIC HEPATITIS C VIRUS?

Andrew Aronsohn, MD; Arjmand R. Mufti, MD, MRCP; and Nancy Reau, MD

After a prolonged course of intensive therapy, the definition of success should be cure. Standard therapy for chronic viral hepatitis C virus (HCV) is 24 to 48 weeks of pegylated interferon in combination with ribavirin, both of which have many potential and often realized side effects. At the end of this therapy, patients want to hear that their HCV has been eradicated and physicians would like to assure them of this result. Yet most clinicians will not be so bold as to label a patient cured of HCV, preferring instead to use the standard terminology sustained virologic response (SVR) or lack of viral replication 6 months after the discontinuation of treatment. What does the word *cure* imply, and how different is this from SVR? Many would consider the end of a medical condition a cure. After the conclusion of therapy, the patient no longer has that particular condition. This is in contrast to a disease that can be controlled but not eliminated. Within the following chapter, we will debate this emotionally charged label and its use in a patient who has successfully completed treatment for HCV.

POINT

Sustained Virologic Response Represents a Cure of Hepatitis C and Long-Term Follow-Up Is Not Necessary

by Andrew Aronsohn, MD

HCV is a leading cause of liver-related morbidity and mortality. SVR, defined as undetectable HCV RNA measured by high sensitivity polymerase chain reaction 24 weeks after

Jensen D.
Controversies in Hepatology: The Experts Analyze Both Sides (pp 73-80)
© 2011 SLACK Incorporated

discontinuation of therapy, has been defined as a virologic cure.[1] Current evidence suggests that SVR is durable, and in a noncirrhotic patient, liver-related complications due to HCV infection are extremely rare, making long-term follow-up unnecessary.

Sustained Virologic Response Is Durable

Patients with SVR remain free of viremia after long-term follow-up. Maylin et al followed 344 patients for a median of 3.27 years and found no patients with detectable serum HCV RNA after achieving SVR.[2] This finding has been supported by a recently described cohort of 150 patients who were followed for 5 years without any evidence of re-emergence of HCV RNA after SVR.[3] Although there have been reports of serologic presence of HCV RNA after SVR, these cases may not represent true relapse of disease.[4,5] Other cases that have been classified as post-SVR "relapse" may, in actuality, be a result of reinfection (notably in patients who continue to be at high risk for exposure), incomplete eradication of the virus during treatment (especially since patients are immune compromised soon after discontinuation of treatment), or a result of higher sensitivity assays detecting viral RNA that remained under the limits of detection using older, less sensitive assays. Given the rarity of reports of post-SVR "relapse" and potential methodological flaws in defining this type of relapse, there is a dearth of evidence that can adequately refute SVR as a virologic cure.

Liver-Related Complications Are Rare Following Sustained Virologic Response

HCV has been shown to cause progression of fibrosis leading to cirrhosis and is a risk factor for hepatocellular carcinoma.[1] The goal of viral eradication is to decrease liver-related complications; this has been well documented. In patients without advanced fibrosis, liver-related complications such as liver failure after SVR are virtually nonexistent.[6] Progression to fibrosis is halted or even reversed after SVR. Toccaceli et al has shown an absence of progression of fibrosis post-SVR, with 43.9% of patients in this cohort showing a histologic improvement in post-SVR biopsies.[7] George et al has supported this finding by failing to demonstrate any increase in fibrosis scores in 37 paired pre- and post-treatment biopsies of patients without advanced liver disease who have achieved SVR.[3] Lack of progression to advanced liver disease after SVR has also been reflected in improved quality of life measurements after successful HCV treatment.[8]

Hepatocellular carcinoma is rare post SVR. Although HCC has been reported after SVR, these cases are most often seen in patients with advanced disease prior to treatment.[9,10] AASLD guidelines advocate for screening for hepatocellular carcinoma in patients with cirrhosis but not in patients with HCV and early-stage fibrosis.[11] Since patients with early stages of liver disease who obtain SVR do not progress to cirrhosis and clinical evidence suggests an extremely low rate of HCC occurrence in the noncirrhotic patient with SVR, regular screening in this patient population cannot be justified.

Hepatitis C Virus Found in Other Tissues Is of No Known Clinical Consequence

Occult HCV infection is defined as HCV RNA found in peripheral blood mononuclear cells or liver tissue in a patient without detectable HCV RNA in the serum.[12] To date, the prevalence of HCV RNA in PBMC and liver tissue in patients post-SVR is not a reproducible finding. Most of the data supporting this notion of occult infection come from a relatively small group of investigators.[2,13-18] No adverse liver-related clinical outcomes have been described in patients with occult HCV infection post-SVR, and there are no currently available data to justify monitoring patients with negative HCV serum RNA levels due to the possibility of occult HCV infection.

Summary

Successful treatment of HCV in a noncirrhotic patient results in sustained eradication of HCV from the serum and a drastic decrease in risk from the sequela of chronic liver diseases such as progression to cirrhosis and hepatocellular carcinoma. Continued patient surveillance in this low-risk population would result in patient anxiety and needless consumption of limited health care resources. SVR in a patient without advanced cirrhosis should be considered a cure that, when achieved, requires no further follow-up.

KEY POINTS

- Late relapse is extremely rare and may be mislabeled reinfection or inaccurate measure of initial viral eradication.
- SVR halts progression to cirrhosis and in some cases may allow regression of fibrosis.
- Hepatocellular carcinoma is rare after SVR in noncirrhotic patients.
- Although occult HCV infection has been demonstrated by some investigators, these findings have never been shown to have clinical significance.
- Clinical consequences are less after SVR; however, long-term follow-up is warranted in cirrhotic patients despite successful HCV therapy.

COUNTERPOINT

Sustained Virologic Response Does Not Represent a Cure of Hepatitis C and Long-Term Follow-Up Is Necessary Under Certain Circumstances

by Arjmand R. Mufti, MD, MRCP

Hepatitis C virus (HCV) is the most common cause of chronic liver disease in the United States, and infection is characterized by a high rate of persistence.[19] Spontaneous remission of the disease is uncommon, and the goal of combination therapy with peginterferon and ribavirin is to prevent complications of hepatitis C. Currently, response to therapy is assessed by measuring serum HCV RNA levels before and after the initiation of therapy. SVR is defined as the absence of HCV RNA from serum by a highly sensitive PCR assay 24 weeks after the discontinuation of therapy.[1] It is abundantly clear that relapse of hepatitis C is rare in the vast majority of patients who have achieved SVR. However, SVR does not represent a true cure of hepatitis C.

Late Virological Relapse After Sustained Virologic Response Is Well Defined

The Oxford English Dictionary defines *cure* as "a complete or permanent remedy," and while the achievement of SVR is vital in mitigating against long-term sequelae of HCV infection, it does not completely protect against a late virological relapse in immune competent persons. Individual trials with interferon monotherapy have revealed late relapse rates of between 4.7% and 9%.[20-22] A meta-analysis by Camma et al of outcomes with interferon monotherapy reported a late virological relapse rate of 8.7%.[23] Following treatment with peginterferon with or without ribavirin, Swain et al reported a late relapse rate of 0.8% after 4 years of follow-up,[24] consistent with data reported independently by other investigators looking at virological relapse with combination therapy.[4] The adoption of therapy with peginterferon and ribavirin as the standard of care has resulted in a significant decrease but not complete eradication of late virological relapse.

Late Virological Response in Immune-Suppressed Patients

HCV is naturally cleared from the body by a T-cell mediated response.[25] Both the innate and adaptive immune responses are involved in this process and result in protective immunity, which is characterized by a mild, limited infection on re-exposure to the virus.[26,27] Combination therapy with peginterferon and ribavirin results in a prolonged inhibition of viral replication. Host immune systems are then able to control the low HCV titres and prevent replication and re-emergence of infection. The achievement of SVR likely represents a state of protective immunity in which serum HCV levels are undetectable with current methods. Indeed, Radkowski et al showed that use of a more sensitive assay such as Reverse Transcription Polymerase Chain Reaction Nucleic Acid Hybridisation (RT-PCR-NAH) demonstrated the presence of the virus in the serum of 4 out of 17 patients, and viral replicative forms were found in lymphocytes of 2 patients and in macrophages of 4 patients.[13]

Furthermore, it is well established that protective immunity can be overcome with immunosuppression. Mehta et al reported the case of a patient who had previously cleared hepatitis C from the serum when he was HIV negative but then developed chronic hepatitis C after a diagnosis of HIV.[28] Re-emergence of HCV in the serum has also been reported after prednisone therapy for bronchitis and after immune suppression postrenal transplantation.[29] The likelihood of reinfection was low as the recurrent viral genotype was identical to the original in both cases. High-risk behavior was not present in either case, and the donor kidney tested negative for hepatitis C.

It is possible that higher viral loads combined with immune suppression result in a loss of SVR as host immunity is no longer capable of controlling viral replication. It therefore follows that recurrence of hepatitis C after liver transplantation is the bane of the hepatologist and is associated with a 23% increase in the rate of death and 30% increase in graft loss compared to patients transplanted for other indications.[30] It has been postulated that excessive immune suppression may perversely exacerbate the post-transplant course in these patients, but this has to be mitigated against the risk of acute rejection.[31] A clear consensus has yet to emerge on the management of these patients and further study is required.

Summary

Successful treatment of HCV in a noncirrhotic patient does indeed result in a durable eradication of HCV from the serum and the achievement of SVR. However, this does not mean that SVR represents a cure where a state of sterilizing immunity is achieved. It likely reflects a setting in which HCV levels are sufficiently suppressed so that they are undetectable in the serum by current conventional PCR methods. This form of protective immunity results in a decrease in the complications of hepatitis C infection, such as progression to cirrhosis and hepatocellular carcinoma. Re-emergence of viremia after immune suppression and data describing late relapse are highly suggestive of a lack of true viral eradication; thus it would be impossible to consider these patients cured and given the significant risk of morbidity and mortality from chronic HCV infection, continued monitoring is indicated.

KEY POINTS

- Newer, more sensitive assays have shown that patients who have achieved SVR still harbor replicative forms of the HCV.

- Although SVR represents a state of protective immunity, it does not mitigate against the development of a late virological relapse.

- Late virological relapse has been shown to occur in both immune competent and immunocompromised patients.

- Given the poor outcome in patients with recurrence of hepatitis C, especially after transplantation, continued monitoring is warranted.

EXPERT OPINION

Sustained Virologic Response Represents a Cure of Hepatitis C Negating the Need for Long-Term Follow-Up

by Nancy Reau, MD

Despite successful therapy, clinicians are hesitant to proclaim a patient cured of hepatitis C. This is certainly based on a combination of logic and emotion. Our experience with other chronic viruses such as human immunodeficiency (HIV) and hepatitis B (HBV) suggests that one is never free from the pathogen despite decades of suppression. Supporting this preconceived notion, HCV RNA has been documented in liver tissue from patients with confirmed SVR.[2] In addition, the presence of HCV has been documented in extrahepatic tissue potentially serving as a reservoir to contribute to relapse after discontinuation of therapy. Little information exists about this phenomenon, let alone any information as to how long or even if HCV can survive and replicate in these locations.[32] In the past, clinicians have been misled into believing an individual cured when technology could not differentiate low levels of virus from undetectable virus, a difference we now realize easily distinguishes a patient at high risk of relapse from potential long-term response. Ultimately, physicians remain hesitant to make any proclamation (positive or negative) without data to support their claim. Fortunately data continue to accumulate in support of long-term viral eradication as a cure from hepatitis C. In a patient without advanced fibrosis, data also support negligible risk for HCV-mediated clinical consequences after SVR, negating the need for long-term follow-up once viral eradication has been documented with a sensitive assay.

Durable long-term viral suppression has now been demonstrated by several large cohorts of patients followed up to 18 years.[2,5,33] Late relapse (beyond 24 weeks after treatment discontinuation) occurred in 0% to 8% of patients followed. When late relapse is observed, it is generally found in association with unusual circumstances resulting in immune suppression close to the end of therapy, such as with chemotherapy or organ transplantation.[29,34,35] Other possible explanations include reinfection, especially if patients resume high-risk behaviors.

Durable viral suppression is actually a surrogate marker for the real goal of therapy: to decrease the risk of clinical consequences. To reiterate Dr. Aronsohn's argument, several large trials with paired histology specimens (pre- and post-treatment) demonstrate stabilization or reversal of hepatic fibrosis, including regression of established cirrhosis in those that achieve SVR.[36,37] Equally important, in those patients that cleared virus only 7% demonstrated a worsening of fibrosis.[38]

Most importantly, along with durable suppression, SVR results in clinical benefits. Patients who clear virus have improved survival and lower incidence of liver-related events such as the development of ascites, hepatic encephalopathy, variceal bleeding, and incidence of HCC.[5,39-42] Even in those with advanced fibrosis, including cirrhosis, improved survival has been shown including a lower rate of liver failure, transplantation, and development of HCC.[6,42] Extrahepatic effects from hepatitis C, including neurologic, hematologic, renal, dermatologic, and glucose intolerance, also tend to improve with successful therapy as do overall quality-of-life measures.[43-47] It is important to remember that those patients with advanced fibrosis (Ishak score 4 to 6) continue to have a risk for hepatic decompensation as well as a risk to develop HCC. Successful therapy only lowers the risk for these life-threatening clinical consequences. Thus despite SVR, regular monitoring and liver cancer screening in this population continues to be warranted for the rest of their lives.

In a patient without advanced liver disease, SVR is a label that effectively represents a cure. This does not imply immunity from reinfection but does equate to durable long to long-term viral suppression virtually eliminating any risk for long term clinical consequences from HCV. If a patient does not have advanced hepatic fibrosis, there is no advantage to continued clinical monitoring.

References

1. Ghany MG, Strader DB, Thomas DL, et al. Diagnosis, management, and treatment of hepatitis C: an update. *Hepatology.* 2009;49(4):1335-1374.
2. Maylin S, Martinot-Peignoux M, Moucari R, et al. Eradication of hepatitis C virus in patients successfully treated for chronic hepatitis C. *Gastroenterology.* 2008;135(3):821-829.
3. George SL, Bacon BR, Brunt EM, et al. Clinical, virologic, histologic, and biochemical outcomes after successful HCV therapy: a 5-year follow-up of 150 patients. *Hepatology.* 2009;49(3):729-738.
4. Desmond CP, Roberts SK, Dudley F, et al. Sustained virological response rates and durability of the response to interferon-based therapies in hepatitis C patients treated in the clinical setting. *J Viral Hepatitis.* 2006;13(5):311-315.
5. Pradat P, Tillmann HL, Sauleda S, et al. Long-term follow-up of the hepatitis C HENCORE cohort: response to therapy and occurrence of liver-related complications. *J Viral Hepatitis.* 2007;14(8):556-563.
6. Veldt BJ, Heathcote EJ, Wedemeyer H, et al. Sustained virologic response and clinical outcomes in patients with chronic hepatitis C and advanced fibrosis. *Ann Intern Med.* 2007;147(10):677-684.
7. Toccaceli F, Laghi V, Capurso L, et al. Long-term liver histology improvement in patients with chronic hepatitis C and sustained response to interferon. *J Viral Hepatitis.* 2003;10(2):126-133.
8. Ware JE Jr., Bayliss MS, Mannocchia M, et al. Health-related quality of life in chronic hepatitis C: impact of disease and treatment response. The Interventional Therapy Group. *Hepatology.* 1999;30(2):550-555.
9. Yu ML, Lin SM, Chuang WL, et al. A sustained virological response to interferon or interferon/ribavirin reduces hepatocellular carcinoma and improves survival in chronic hepatitis C: a nationwide, multicentre study in Taiwan. *Antiviral Ther.* 2006;11(8):985-994.
10. Kobayashi S, Takeda T, Enomoto M, et al. Development of hepatocellular carcinoma in patients with chronic hepatitis C who had a sustained virological response to interferon therapy: a multicenter, retrospective cohort study of 1124 patients. *Liver Int.* 2007;27(2):186-191.
11. Bruix J, Sherman M. Management of hepatocellular carcinoma. *Hepatology.* 2005;42(5):1208-1236.
12. Carreno V. Occult hepatitis C virus infection: a new form of hepatitis C. *World J Gastroenterol.* 2006;12(43):6922-6925.
13. Radkowski M, Gallegos-Orozco JF, Jablonska J, et al. Persistence of hepatitis C virus in patients successfully treated for chronic hepatitis C. *Hepatology.* 2005;41(1):106-114.
14. Carreno V, Pardo M, Lopez-Alcorocho JM, et al. Detection of hepatitis C virus (HCV) RNA in the liver of healthy, anti-HCV antibody-positive, serum HCV RNA-negative patients with normal alanine aminotransferase levels. *J Infect Dis.* 2006;194(1):53-60.
15. Castillo I, Rodriguez-Inigo E, Lopez-Alcorocho JM, et al. Hepatitis C virus replicates in the liver of patients who have a sustained response to antiviral treatment. *Clin Infect Dis.* 2006;43(10):1277-1283.
16. Castillo I, Rodriguez-Inigo E, Bartolome J, et al. Hepatitis C virus replicates in peripheral blood mononuclear cells of patients with occult hepatitis C virus infection. *Gut.* 2005;54(5):682-685.
17. De Mitri MS, Morsica G, Chen CH, et al. Complete eradication of hepatitis C virus after interferon treatment for chronic hepatitis C. *J Gastroenterol Hepatol.* 1997;29(3):255-261.
18. Romeo R, Pol S, Berthelot P, et al. Eradication of hepatitis C virus RNA after alpha-interferon therapy. *Ann Intern Med.* 1994;121(4):276-277.
19. National Institutes of Health Consensus Development Conference Statement: Management of hepatitis C 2002. *Gastroenterol.* 2002;123(6):2082-2099.
20. Veldt BJ, Saracco G, Boyer N, et al. Long-term clinical outcome of chronic hepatitis C patients with sustained virological response to interferon monotherapy. *Gut.* 2004;53(10):1504-1508.
21. Reichard O, Glaumann H, Fryden A, et al. Long-term follow-up of chronic hepatitis C patients with sustained virological response to alpha-interferon. *J Hepatol.* 1999;30(5):783-787.
22. Khokhar N. Late relapse in chronic hepatitis C after sustained viral response to interferon and ribavirin. *J Gastroenterol Hepatol.* 2004;19(4):471-472.
23. Camma C, Di Marco V, Lo Iacono O, et al. Long-term course of interferon-treated chronic hepatitis C. *J Hepatol.* 1998;28(4):531-537.
24. Swain M, Lai M-Y, Shiffman ML, et al. Treatment of patients with chronic hepatitis C (CHC) with peginterferon alfa-2a (40KD) (Pegasys) alone or in combination with ribavirin (copegus) results in long-lasting sustained virological response. *J Hepatol.* 2003;38(Suppl2):175.
25. Lauer GM, Barnes E, Lucas M, et al. High resolution analysis of cellular immune responses in resolved and persistent hepatitis C virus infection. *Gastroenterol.* 2004;127(3):924-936.
26. Bassett SE, Guerra B, Brasky K, et al. Protective immune response to hepatitis C virus in chimpanzees rechallenged following clearance of primary infection. *Hepatol.* 2001;33(6):1479-1487.

27. Nascimbeni M, Mizukoshi E, Bosmann M, et al. Kinetics of CD4+ and CD8+ memory T-cell responses during hepatitis C virus rechallenge of previously recovered chimpanzees. *J Virol.* 2003;77(8):4781-4793.

28. Mehta SH, Cox A, Hoover DR, et al. Protection against persistence of hepatitis C. *Lancet.* 2002;359(9316):1478-1483.

29. Lin A, Thadareddy A, Goldstein MJ, et al. Immune suppression leading to hepatitis C virus re-emergence after sustained virological response. *J Med Virology.* 2008;80(10):1720-1722.

30. Forman LM, Lewis JD, Berlin JA, et al. The association between hepatitis C infection and survival after orthotopic liver transplantation. *Gastroenterol.* 2002;122(4):889-896.

31. Berenguer M. What determines the natural history of recurrent hepatitis C after liver transplantation? *J Hepatol.* 2005;42(4):448-456.

32. de Almeida PR, de Mattos AA, Amaral KM, et al. Treatment of hepatitis C with peginterferon and ribavirin in a public health program. *Hepato-Gastroenterol.* 2009;56(89):223-226.

33. Lindsay K, Manns M, Gordon S, et al. Clearance of HCV at 5 year follow-up for peginterferon alfa-2b ± ribavirin is predicted by sustained virologic response at 24 weeks post treatment. In: DDW. San Diego, California; 2008.

34. Thomopoulos K, Giannakoulas NC, Tsamandas AC, et al. Recurrence of HCV infection in a sustained responder after chemotherapy for non-Hodgkin's lymphoma: successful retreatment. *Am J Med Sci.* 2008;336(1):73-76.

35. Everson GT, Trotter J, Forman L, et al. Treatment of advanced hepatitis C with a low accelerating dosage regimen of antiviral therapy. *Hepatol.* 2005;42(2):255-262.

36. Manns MP, McHutchison JG, Gordon SC, et al. Peginterferon alfa-2b plus ribavirin compared with interferon alfa-2b plus ribavirin for initial treatment of chronic hepatitis C: a randomised trial. *Lancet.* 2001;358(9286):958-965.

37. Poynard T, Bedossa P, Chevallier M, et al. A comparison of three interferon alfa-2b regimens for the long-term treatment of chronic non-A, non-B hepatitis. Multicenter Study Group. *N Engl J Med.* 1995;332(22):1457-1462.

38. Poynard T, McHutchison J, Manns M, et al. Impact of pegylated interferon alfa-2b and ribavirin on liver fibrosis in patients with chronic hepatitis C. *Gastroenterol.* 2002;122(5):1303-1313.

39. Bruno S, Stroffolini T, Colombo M, et al. Sustained virological response to interferon-alpha is associated with improved outcome in HCV-related cirrhosis: a retrospective study. *Hepatology.* 2007;45(3):579-587.

40. Braks RE, Ganne-Carrie N, Fontaine H, et al. Effect of sustained virological response on long-term clinical outcome in 113 patients with compensated hepatitis C-related cirrhosis treated by interferon alpha and ribavirin. *World J Gastroenterol.* 2007;13(42):5648-5653.

41. Alonso S, Rincón D, Bárcena.R., et al. Effect of sustained virological response to pedinterferon plus ribavirin therpay on liver related free survival in HCV cirrhotic patients: factors predicting virological response. *Hepatology.* 2008;48(4Suppl):1298A.

42. Cardoso AF, Moucari R, Giuily N, et al. Lower risk of hepatocellular carcinoma and improved survival in patients with HCV related cirrhosis with sustained virological response. *Hepatology.* 2008;48(4Suppl):264A.

43. Calleja JL, Albillos A, Moreno-Otero R, et al. Sustained response to interferon-alpha or to interferon-alpha plus ribavirin in hepatitis C virus-associated symptomatic mixed cryoglobulinaemia. *Aliment Pharmacol Ther.* 1999;13(9):1179-1186.

44. Rossi P, Bertani T, Baio P, et al. Hepatitis C virus-related cryoglobulinemic glomerulonephritis: long-term remission after antiviral therapy. *Kidney Int.* 2003;63(6):2236-2241.

45. Loustaud-Ratti V, Liozon E, Karaaslan H, et al. Interferon alpha and ribavirin for membranoproliferative glomerulonephritis and hepatitis C infection. *Am J Med.* 2002;113(6):516-519.

46. Misiani R, Bellavita P, Baio P, et al. Successful treatment of HCV-associated cryoglobulinaemic glomerulonephritis with a combination of interferon-alpha and ribavirin. *Nephrol Dial Transplant.* 1999;14(6):1558-1560.

47. Simo R, Lecube A, Genesca J, et al. Sustained virological response correlates with reduction in the incidence of glucose abnormalities in patients with chronic hepatitis C virus infection. *Diabetes Care.* 2006;29(11):2462-2466.

SECTION III
LIVER TUMORS

SHOULD LIVING DONOR LIVER TRANSPLANTATION BE AN OPTION FOR PATIENTS WITH HEPATOCELLULAR CARCINOMA BEYOND THE MILAN CRITERIA?

Brett E. Fortune, MD; Alvaro Martinez-Camacho, MD; and James R. Burton Jr, MD

Hepatocellular carcinoma (HCC) is one of the leading causes of death worldwide. In the setting of end-stage liver disease, liver transplantation (LT) is the only definitive therapy. With careful patient selection, LT for HCC has achieved survival rates comparable to those of non-malignant liver disease. Given the current scarcity of available deceased donor organs, living donor liver transplantation (LDLT) has become an option for managing patients with HCC, one that required balance between benefit to recipient and risk to the donor.

POINT

Living Donor Liver Transplantation Is a Viable Option for Patients Who Are Beyond Milan Criteria

by Brett E. Fortune, MD

LT is the preferred treatment strategy for unresectable HCC. The landmark paper by Mazzaferro et al illustrated that carefully selected patients with HCC could achieve a survival rate equivalent to patients transplanted without HCC (75% survival at 4 years).[1] The Mazzaferro (Milan) criteria

Jensen D.
*Controversies in Hepatology: The Experts Analyze Both
Sides (pp 83-92)*
© 2011 SLACK Incorporated

Table 9-1.		
TUMOR CHARACTERISTICS OF HEPATOCELLULAR CARCINOMA DEFINING MILAN AND UNIVERSITY OF CALIFORNIA, SAN FRANCISCO CRITERIA FOR LIVER TRANSPLANTATION		
	MILAN CRITERIA	UNIVERSITY OF CALIFORNIA, SAN FRANCISCO CRITERIA
One tumor	<5 cm	≤6.5 cm
Two or three tumors	All tumors <3 cm	Largest tumor ≤4.5 cm and total tumor diameter ≤8 cm
No evidence of metastases or gross vascular invasion. Size refers to diameter of tumor as measured on cross sectional imaging.		

(Table 9-1) have since been adopted by the United Network for Organ Sharing (UNOS) in the United States to assign a higher priority for a patient with HCC awaiting liver transplantation. However, applying restrictive criteria such as the Milan criteria may exclude patients with HCC at various advanced stages who may potentially benefit from LT. This has led to careful expansion of criteria with similar outcomes as the Milan criteria (University of California, San Francisco [UCSF] criteria; see Table 9-1).[2] For some patients, living donor liver transplantation (LDLT) may offer the only chance at long-term survival.

Benefits of Living Donor Liver Transplantation

LDLT has several potential benefits regardless of indication. Due to being an elective, scheduled procedure, LDLT results in shorter wait times, potentially reducing death or being removed from the wait list from complications of liver disease or tumor progression. In addition, given that demand for donor organs far exceeds the supply of organs, LDLT expands the donor pool. Finally and most importantly, after many years of perfecting the procedure and gaining experience in donor selection, LDLT has achieved overall similar survival rates when compared to deceased donor liver transplantation (DDLT).[3-6]

Potential Benefits of Living Donor Liver Transplantation in Patients Beyond Milan Criteria But Within University of California, San Francisco Criteria

Two analyses show that LDLT is superior to DDLT for those with HCC within Milan criteria when waiting times for deceased donor organs exceed 6 months.[7,8] When tumors exceed Milan criteria, some studies have observed increased tumor recurrence rates as well as lower overall survival rates after LDLT.[9-11] However, when LDLT is limited to UCSF criteria survival rates, LDLT and DDLT are equivalent.[2,10,12-14] Hwang et al performed a retrospective multicenter analysis of 216 patients who received LDLT for HCC.[10] Three-year survival for those meeting Milan criteria (n = 151) was 91%, similar for those meeting the UCSF criteria (n = 167) at 91%. With expanding criteria to the UCSF criteria, an additional 16 patients (7.4% of the total sample size) were transplanted without significant compromise in overall survival. Other studies using the UCSF criteria reveal similar findings.[12,13,15] Based on these results, it appears that LDLT for HCC within UCSF criteria can achieve acceptable outcomes.

Potential Benefits of Living Donor Liver Transplantation in Patients Beyond University of California, San Francisco Criteria

The past decade has seen several advances in pharmacological and locoregional therapies for the management of patients with unresectable HCC beyond Milan criteria. Although these advances, especially in combination, do provide some survival benefit (17% to 50% 3-year survival), outcome varies based on extent of tumor burden and the patients' hepatic reserve.[16-18]

Another consideration for patients who exceed Milan criteria at diagnosis of HCC is to "downstage" tumors to within Milan criteria with locoregional therapy before considering LT. Outcomes with this approach are similar to that of transplanting patients within Milan criteria.[19,20] Downstaging likely does not change tumor biology, but rather extends the time from diagnosis to LT, identifying slowly growing tumors more appropriate for transplantation. Patients with decompensated liver disease and extensive HCC who exceed Milan (and UCSF) criteria are often not candidates for locoregional therapy and their only option would be LDLT to resolve both their failing liver and HCC. Based on studies using UCSF criteria, even patients beyond UCSF criteria demonstrate a 3-year survival rate greater than 50%.[10,12,13] Compared to mortality of 100% without LT, from a recipient standpoint the benefits of LDLT appear clear.

Mazzaferro et al recently developed a model to predict survival probabilities in patients beyond Milan criteria based on objective tumor characteristics such as tumor size, number of tumors, and presence of microscopic vascular invasion.[21] This study included 1556 patients transplanted for HCC at 36 centers with 1112 patients exceeding Milan criteria on post-LT pathology review. In the group exceeding Milan criteria, the largest tumor was 4 cm (0.4 to 20 cm) and the median number of nodules was 4 (1 to 20). Forty-one percent had microscopic vascular invasion. The overall 5-year survival rate for those exceeding Milan was 53.6% (95% CI, 50.1% to 57%) compared to 73.3% (95% CI, 68.2% to 77.7%) for those within Milan criteria. A subgroup, in the absence of vascular invasion, fulfilled the so-called "up to 7 criteria," with 7 being the result of the sum of the size (in cm) and number of tumors for any given HCC (ie, 1 nodule up to 6 cm in size [1 + 6 = 7], 2 nodules up to 5 cm in size [2 + 5 = 7], 3 nodules up to 4 cm in size [3 + 4 = 7], or 5 tumors up to 2 cm in size [5 + 2 = 7]).[21] Five-year survival in this group of 283 patients was 71.2% (95% CI, 64.3% to 77.0%), which was not significantly different from the overall 5-year survival rate for 444 patients (73.3%) with HCC within Milan criteria, irrespective of microvascular invasion (68.2% to 77.7%). This may be a useful tool when considering LDLT for HCC by addressing the need to balance patients' expected outcomes with risk to a donor.

Summary and Future Directions

LDLT has been successful in expanding the donor pool to reduce the number of patients dying on the waiting list. LDLT for HCC within Milan criteria has similar survival rates when compared to DDLT. Furthermore, LDLT offers the only option for patients outside of Milan criteria who are not candidates for locoregional therapy on account of decompensated liver disease. LDLT will need to be constantly evaluated to ensure that the fine ethical line of recipient benefit does not abuse the risk to donors. The transplant community must continue to review the data of recipient and donor outcomes to ensure that this practice is indeed beneficial to the health care system. LDLT is viable for patients with HCC no matter what criteria you use as long as macrovascular invasion or metastases are not present.

KEY POINTS

- Equivalent survival to DDLT if within UCSF criteria.
- Only life-saving option in patients with decompensated liver disease.
- Better survival than palliative measures.

COUNTERPOINT

Living Donor Liver Transplantation for Hepatocellular Carcinoma Exceeding Milan Criteria Is Not Ready for Prime-Time Use

by Alvaro Martinez-Camacho, MD

Hepatocellular carcinoma (HCC) is a common cancer worldwide with an estimated 632,000 cases identified annually.[22] Furthermore, the incidence of HCC has steadily risen within the United States.[23] Cirrhosis secondary to chronic liver disease is the most common risk factor for HCC.[24] Liver transplantation is not only potentially curative for HCC but also for end-stage liver disease.[25] Consequently, the United Network for Organ Sharing adopted criteria to determine priority for transplanting patients with HCC based on the Milan criteria (Table 9-1), which provides excellent overall and disease-free survival (Table 9-2).[1] However, given a limited donor pool, waiting times can be prolonged and lead to removal of up to 18% of potential recipients from the wait list due to tumor progression or death.[26] As a result, LDLT has become an important alternative to DDLT in many countries.[4,27]

Data Supporting Living Donor Liver Transplantation for Hepatocellular Carcinoma Are Heterogeneous and Yield Mixed Results

Studies of LDLT for HCC report mixed results with overall survival ranging from 48% to 77% (Table 9-3). Researchers designed these studies to evaluate outcomes of LDLT for HCC, but included a heterogeneous group of tumors (range 20% to 67% exceeding Milan criteria),[9,13,28-30] making direct comparison of outcomes difficult. Common findings include shorter waiting time to transplantation and increased recurrence of tumor (4% to 43%) compared to DDLT. Importantly, a large multicenter study of LDLT reported a significantly higher rate of tumor recurrence (36.6%) with associated lower overall and disease-free survival (60.4% and 52.6%, respectively) 3 years after LDLT for HCC exceeding Milan criteria compared to HCC within Milan criteria (78.7% and 79.1%, respectively).[9]

Two important conclusions are reached from the studies above. First, shorter waiting times with LDLT prevent identification of biologically aggressive tumors (so-called "fast-track

Table 9-2.

RESULTS FROM DECEASED DONOR LIVER TRANSPLANTATION FOR HEPATOCELLULAR CARCINOMA STRATIFIED BY TUMOR CHARACTERISTIC

	EXCEEDING MILAN CRITERIA[1]	EXCEEDING MILAN CRITERIA[1]	EXCEEDING UCSF CRITERIA[2]
Overall survival	75%	50%	75%
Disease-free survival	83%	59%	81%
Tumor recurrence	8%	23%	8%

effect"). Tumor behavior is important because cancers have diverse genetics associated with differing rates of growth, vascular invasion, and recurrence.[31-33] Second, the technique of LDLT requires significant center experience before outcomes are comparable to DDLT and may be a suboptimal cancer surgery, as suggested by the A2ALL group.[4,29]

Increased Tumor Recurrence After Living Donor Liver Transplantation for Hepatocellular Carcinoma Exceeding Milan Criteria

Most data specifically evaluating LDLT for HCC exceeding Milan criteria are limited to single-center case series. One study of 22 LDLT recipients with tumor exceeding UCSF criteria reported significantly reduced overall and disease-free survival (62% and 34%, respectively) at 3 years due to a high recurrence rate of 32%.[34] Another center found patients exceeding Milan criteria had reduced survival at 3 years (68.6%) compared to patients within Milan criteria (88.4%), which likely was attributable to HCC recurrences limited to the former group.[13] This group

Table 9-3.

RECENT STUDIES REPORTING RESULTS OF LIVING DONOR LIVER TRANSPLANTATION FOR HEPATOCELLULAR CARCINOMA AT 3-YEARS POST-TRANSPLANTATION

AUTHOR	NUMBER OF PATIENTS	OVERALL PATIENT SURVIVAL	DISEASE-FREE SURVIVAL	RECURRENCE RATE
Fisher[29]	58	67%	58%	29%
Todo[9]	316	69%	65%	13%
Di Sandro[28]	25	77%	96%	4%
Fouzas[34]	22*	62%*	34%*	32%*
Soejima[13]	60	69%	74%*	14%
Woo[35]	37*	48%*	55%*	43%*
Ito[30]	125	68%**	N/A	16%**

*Results reported for recipients with tumor exceeding Milan criteria. **Results reported at 5 years post-transplantation.

also reported that a pre-LT tumor diameter >5 cm independently predicted worse outcomes. Another analysis over 10 years from 37 recipients of LDLT for HCC exceeding Milan criteria reported a very high recurrence rate of 55% within 3 years.[35] Interestingly, poor prognostic markers included tumors >6 cm in diameter, tumors exposed to liver surface, and progressive tumors despite pre-LT locoregional therapy. Another center retrospectively identified 125 cases of LDLT for HCC and demonstrated that tumor recurrence was significantly higher in cases of tumor exceeding Milan criteria (34.3%) compared to those within Milan criteria (9.7%) upon initial analysis.[30] After multivariate analysis of risk factors for recurrence using pre-LT variables, they demonstrated that patients with no more than 10 nodules all <5 cm in diameter and a protein induced by vitamin K antagonist-II (PIVKA-II) level less than 400 mAU/mL had a 5-year overall survival and recurrence rate of 86.7% and 4.9%, respectively, compared to 34.4% and 60.5%, respectively, for patients outside these criteria. However, most centers cannot routinely measure PIVKA-II. Moreover, prospective studies to validate these new criteria are needed before they can be applied to regular practice.

Dilemmas Unique to Living Donor Liver Transplantation

Potential morbidity to the donor is unique to LDLT compared to DDLT. Partial donor hepatectomy is a complex procedure with not insignificant risk and recovery time. Postoperative complications (biliary and wound infections) occur in up to 35% of donors and mortality is estimated at 0.8%.[36] Furthermore, while recent survey studies demonstrated that donors perceive a psychological benefit after donation, others show up to 20% of donors experienced an unexpected significant financial burden after donation.[37,38]

Several ethical questions are encountered when LDLT is performed for HCC outside of Milan criteria.[39,40] What is considered acceptable overall and disease-free survival after LDLT for HCC, and is it acceptable to use lower cutoffs than what is expected for DDLT? Who (donor, recipient, or transplant team) should decide whether the benefit of LDLT for HCC outside Milan criteria outweighs the potential increased risk of recurrence after transplantation and risk to a donor? Should recipients, who presumably were excluded for DDLT due to tumor burden, that experience primary graft nonfunction be emergently re-listed for a deceased donor allograft? These and other unforeseen issues should be addressed before routinely using LDLT for HCC exceeding Milan criteria.

KEY POINTS

- Lower overall survival in patients exceeding Milan criteria.
- Higher rate of tumor recurrence.
- Shortened wait times do not allow for adequate monitoring of tumor biology.
- Potential risk to living donor.
- Ethical considerations, including primary graft nonfunction.

EXPERT OPINION

Living Donor Liver Transplantation Is an Acceptable Option for Recipients Exceeding Milan Criteria With Careful Recipient Selection

by James R. Burton Jr, MD

The demand for LT has and will always exceed the supply of donor organs. The transplant community has an obligation to balance the competing demands of equity, justice, and benefit. The current allocation of donor livers to patients with HCC (Milan criteria) ensures effective use of a scarce resource as well as equity of access. Few options with transplantation exist to achieve a potential cure for patients with HCC outside Milan criteria. One option is utilizing a cadaveric organ, which requires individual appeals to regional review boards for priority points based on fulfilling UCSF criteria[2] or successfully undergoing downstaging protocols.[20] The other option is LDLT where rules are not dictated by graft shortage and waiting lists, but rather weighing a balance between benefit to recipient and risk to the donor.

To date, there are no convincing data that the regenerating liver in LDLT increases risk of recurrent HCC. After adjusting for tumor characteristics, it appears that LDLT is equivalent to DDLT for treating HCC. The landmark paper by Mazzaferro (Milan criteria) showed that post-LT outcome could be predicted by size and number of tumors.[1] However, size and number of tumors are only surrogates of cancer biological behavior. Histological and molecular information about tumors may provide very important information about recurrence. However, performing liver biopsy of HCC is not routinely done in clinical practice on account of a risk—admittedly low—of needle tract spread of tumor. Until the use of molecular markers is validated, we are currently left with size and number of tumors as the only determinant of risk for recurrent disease after transplantation.

Mazzaferro has made another important contribution to the utilization of LT for HCC with the development of a model for patients exceeding Milan criteria based on objective tumor characteristics (again size and number) to provide individual survival estimates.[21] A by-product tool of this analysis was the "Metroticket Calculator," an easy-to-use utility available online that can calculate 3- and 5-year overall survival probabilities with confidence intervals on the basis of maximum tumor size and number. A worse case survival prediction can also be determined based on the presence of vascular invasion from explant analysis. By no means perfect, this model does have a number of obvious limitations. Patients in this study were a highly selected group outside Milan criteria, so an obvious selection bias exists. Additionally, data about tumor characteristics were based on explant information, not pre-LT imaging assessment. It is well known that imaging can understage tumor burden in the explant.[41] Nonetheless, Metroticket is a useful tool in considering LDLT for HCC by addressing the balance of recipient outcome to weigh against donor risk.

Since a donor organ is not being taken out of the donor pool, we should expand the criteria to which we offer LDLT for HCC. Applying restrictive criteria such as the Milan criteria may exclude patients with HCC from a potentially life-saving procedure. There is no doubt that LDLT saves lives. However, we have learned that LDLT is not without significant risk to the donor even in the hands of experienced surgeons and programs. The role of LDLT in HCC (and other indications for LT) is analogous to running into a burning building to save a loved one. Potential donors may disregard the warnings not to run into such a building only concerned with saving a recipient's life. In most cases, potential donors make their decision to donate before any information of risks is acquired. Without clear understanding of donor risk, it is difficult to address the question of what is an acceptable 3- or 5-year survival after LDLT for HCC. This risk/benefit assessment is not only one that needs to be done by the potential donor (as well as recipient), but by the surgical team as well. There are not many single therapies for terminal cancer that offer a chance for cure, like LDLT has the potential to offer for recipients with HCC. With further research into donor risks and better means of predicting recurrence after LT, I am confident that we will find there is a clear benefit to offering LDLT to patients outside Milan criteria.

References

1.   Mazzaferro V, Regalia E, Doci R, et al. Liver transplantation for the treatment of small hepatocellular carcinomas in patients with cirrhosis. *N Engl J Med*. 1996;334:693-699.
2.   Yao FY, Ferrell L, Bass NM, et al. Liver transplantation for hepatocellular carcinoma: expansion of the tumor size limits does not adversely impact survival. *Hepatology*. 2001;33:1394-1403.
3.   Liu CL, Fan ST, Lo CM, et al. Operative outcomes of adult-to-adult right lobe live donor liver transplantation: a comparative study with cadaveric whole-graft liver transplantation in a single center. *Ann Surg*. 2006;243:404-410.
4.   Olthoff KM, Merion RM, Ghobrial RM, et al. Outcomes of 385 adult-to-adult living donor liver transplant recipients: a report from the A2ALL Consortium. *Ann Surg*. 2005;242:314-323.
5.   Berg CL, Gillespie BW, Merion RM, et al. Improvement in survival associated with adult-to-adult living donor liver transplantation. *Gastroenterology*. 2007;133:1806-1813.
6.   Maluf DG, Stravitz RT, Cotterell AH, et al. Adult living donor versus deceased donor liver transplantation: a 6-year single center experience. *Am J Transplant*. 2005;5:149-156.
7.   Sarasin FP, Majno PE, Llovet JM, et al. Living donor liver transplantation for early hepatocellular carcinoma: a life-expectancy and cost-effectiveness perspective. *Hepatology*. 2001;33:1073-1079.
8.   Cheng SJ, Pratt DS, Freeman RB Jr, et al. Living-donor versus cadaveric liver transplantation for non-resectable small hepatocellular carcinoma and compensated cirrhosis: a decision analysis. *Transplantation*. 2001;72:861-868.
9.   Todo S, Furukawa H. Living donor liver transplantation for adult patients with hepatocellular carcinoma: experience in Japan. *Ann Surg*. 2004;240:451-459.
10. Hwang S, Lee SG, Joh JW, et al. Liver transplantation for adult patients with hepatocellular carcinoma in Korea: comparison between cadaveric donor and living donor liver transplantations. *Liver Transpl*. 2005;11:1265-1272.
11. Takada Y, Ueda M, Ito T, et al. Living donor liver transplantation as a second-line therapeutic strategy for patients with hepatocellular carcinoma. *Liver Transpl*. 2006;12:912-919.
12. Jonas S, Mittler J, Pascher A, et al. Living donor liver transplantation of the right lobe for hepatocellular carcinoma in cirrhosis in a European center. *Liver Transpl*. 2007;13:896-903.
13. Soejima Y, Taketomi A, Yoshizumi T, et al. Extended indication for living donor liver transplantation in patients with hepatocellular carcinoma. *Transplantation*. 2007;83:893-899.
14. Yao FY, Xiao L, Bass NM, et al. Liver transplantation for hepatocellular carcinoma: validation of the UCSF-expanded criteria based on preoperative imaging. *Am J Transplant*. 2007;7:2587-2596.
15. Vakili K, Pomposelli JJ, Cheah YL, et al. Living donor liver transplantation for hepatocellular carcinoma: increased recurrence but improved survival. *Liver Transpl*. 2009;15:1861-1866.
16. Lencioni R. Loco-regional treatment of hepatocellular carcinoma. *Hepatology*. 2010;52:762-773.
17. Llovet JM, Ricci S, Mazzaferro V, et al. Sorafenib in advanced hepatocellular carcinoma. *N Engl J Med*. 2008;359:378-390.
18. Wang W, Shi J, Xie WF. Transarterial chemoembolization in combination with percutaneous ablation therapy in unresectable hepatocellular carcinoma: a meta-analysis. *Liver Int*. 2010;30:741-749.
19. Yao FY, Hirose R, LaBerge JM, et al. A prospective study on downstaging of hepatocellular carcinoma prior to liver transplantation. *Liver Transpl*. 2005;11:1505-1514.

20. Yao FY, Kerlan RK, Jr., Hirose R, et al. Excellent outcome following down-staging of hepatocellular carcinoma prior to liver transplantation: an intention-to-treat analysis. *Hepatology.* 2008;48:819-827.

21. Mazzaferro V, Llovet JM, Miceli R, et al. Predicting survival after liver transplantation in patients with hepatocellular carcinoma beyond the Milan criteria: a retrospective, exploratory analysis. *Lancet Oncol.* 2009;10:35-43.

22. Mathers C, Fat DM, et al. The global burden of disease: 2004 update. Geneva, Switzerland: World Health Organization; 2008.

23. El-Serag HB, Davila JA, Petersen NJ, et al. The continuing increase in the incidence of hepatocellular carcinoma in the United States: an update. *Ann Intern Med.* 2003;139:817-823.

24. Bruix J, Sherman M, Llovet JM, et al. Clinical management of hepatocellular carcinoma. Conclusions of the Barcelona-2000 EASL conference. European Association for the Study of the Liver. *J Hepatol.* 2001;35:421-430.

25. Bruix J, Sherman M. Management of hepatocellular carcinoma. *Hepatology.* 2005;42:1208-1236.

26. Pelletier SJ, Fu S, Thyagarajan V, et al. An intention-to-treat analysis of liver transplantation for hepatocellular carcinoma using organ procurement transplant network data. *Liver Transpl.* 2009;15:859-868.

27. Jeon H, Lee SG. Living donor liver transplantation. *Curr Opin Organ Transplant.* 2010;15:283-287.

28. Di Sandro S, Slim AO, Giacomoni A, et al. Living donor liver transplantation for hepatocellular carcinoma: long-term results compared with deceased donor liver transplantation. *Transplant Proc.* 2009;41:1283-1285.

29. Fisher RA, Kulik LM, Freise CE, et al. Hepatocellular carcinoma recurrence and death following living and deceased donor liver transplantation. *Am J Transplant.* 2007;7:1601-1608.

30. Ito T, Takada Y, Ueda M, et al. Expansion of selection criteria for patients with hepatocellular carcinoma in living donor liver transplantation. *Liver Transpl.* 2007;13:1637-1644.

31. Laurent-Puig P, Legoix P, Bluteau O, et al. Genetic alterations associated with hepatocellular carcinomas define distinct pathways of hepatocarcinogenesis. *Gastroenterology.* 2001;120:1763-1773.

32. Laurent-Puig P, Zucman-Rossi J. Genetics of hepatocellular tumors. *Oncogene.* 2006;25:3778-3786.

33. Budhu A, Forgues M, Ye QH, et al. Prediction of venous metastases, recurrence, and prognosis in hepatocellular carcinoma based on a unique immune response signature of the liver microenvironment. *Cancer Cell.* 2006;10:99-111.

34. Fouzas I, Sotiropoulos GC, Lang H, et al. Living donor liver transplantation for hepatocellular carcinoma in patients exceeding the UCSF criteria. *Transplant Proc.* 2008;40:3185-3188.

35. Woo HY, Jang JW, Choi JY, et al. Living donor liver transplantation in hepatocellular carcinoma beyond the Milan criteria. *Liver Int.* 2008;28:1120-1128.

36. Ghobrial RM, Freise CE, Trotter JF, et al. Donor morbidity after living donation for liver transplantation. *Gastroenterology.* 2008;135:468-476.

37. Holtzman S, Adcock L, Dubay DA, et al. Financial, vocational, and interpersonal impact of living liver donation. *Liver Transpl.* 2009;15:1435-1442.

38. Schulz KH, Kroencke S, Beckmann M, et al. Mental and physical quality of life in actual living liver donors versus potential living liver donors: a prospective, controlled, multicenter study. *Liver Transpl.* 2009;15:1676-1687.

39. Lee HS. Liver transplantation for hepatocellular carcinoma beyond the Milan criteria: the controversies continue. *Dig Dis.* 2007;25:296-298.

40. Volk ML, Marrero JA, Lok AS, Ubel PA. Who decides? Living donor liver transplantation for advanced hepatocellular carcinoma. *Transplantation.* 2006;82:1136-1139.

41. Yao FY. Liver transplantation for hepatocellular carcinoma: beyond the Milan criteria. *Am J Transplant.* 2008;8:1982-1989.

RESECT OR OBSERVE ASYMPTOMATIC HEPATIC ADENOMA?

Joseph Ahn, MD, MS; Anjana Pillai, MD; and Stanley Martin Cohen, MD

Hepatic adenomas are uncommon liver tumors generally found in women. Although the majority of these tumors follow a benign course, there can be complications including rupture, hemorrhage, and malignant transformation. These complications correlate with tumor size.

While most experts would advocate a surgical approach to patients with symptomatic hepatic adenomas, the management of asymptomatic hepatic adenomas is quite controversial. This chapter will address this controversy and evaluate the data for resection versus observation of the asymptomatic hepatic adenoma. The chapter will conclude with a summary of the opposing viewpoints as well as a suggested approach to these patients.

POINT

Resect Asymptomatic Hepatic Adenomas

by Joseph Ahn, MD, MS

Since the 1960s the frequency, size, and number of reported hepatic adenomas has increased, which can be attributed to the increased use of oral contraceptives (OCPs) and anabolic steroids. In addition, the improved ability of imaging studies to detect small lesions, along with an increase in imaging utilization, has led to a growing number of asymptomatic hepatic adenomas discovered.

Jensen D.
Controversies in Hepatology: The Experts Analyze Both Sides (pp 93-100)
© 2011 SLACK Incorporated

The controversy in management of asymptomatic hepatic adenomas reflects a lack of randomized controlled trials, as outlined in a recent Cochrane database review.[1] What is not controversial is the increased risk of hepatic adenomas to rupture, hemorrhage, and progress to malignancy.

The risk of rupture and hemorrhage increases with increasing lesion size, usually once the diameter reaches 4 to 5 cm. In 2 of the largest series of 122 patients and 124 patients, up to 25% presented with a rupture associated with an increase in size.[2,3] This association of size with rupture and bleeding was supported in multiple reports which found a 25% to 40% presentation with rupture and hemorrhage.[4-7] An increase in the number of lesions, a subcapsular or peripheral location of the lesions, and use of high-dose OCPs were additional risk factors for rupture. As most hepatic adenomas do not have a fibrous capsule, rupture may lead to hemorrhage. In addition, an asymptomatic initial presentation was not protective of progression to rupture or hemorrhage. More importantly, inaction to resect asymptomatic hepatic adenomas may leave patients facing a mortality risk of 5% to 20% if they later present with an unexpected rupture and hemorrhage requiring emergent surgical intervention, especially during pregnancy.[5,8]

Asymptomatic hepatic adenomas also remain at risk for malignant degeneration or transformation to hepatocellular carcinoma, which can occur in 4% to 13% of patients.[2,3,5,6,9-11] This risk of malignant transformation increases with adenomas >5 cm.[2,3]

Although opting to observe asymptomatic hepatic adenomas, especially after discontinuation of OCPs, in the hope of regression or reduction in size appears reasonable on initial consideration, data are mixed on the success of this approach. Reports of significant regression are counter-balanced by reports of persistence and progression.[8,11-14] More concerning are reports of malignant transformation in asymptomatic hepatic adenomas, even after a decrease in size or disappearance after OCP discontinuation.[15] Thus, although monitoring the patient off OCPs and steroids appears reasonable, it cannot be unequivocally relied upon to attenuate the risk of complications. These findings support the recommendation to resect all adenomas regardless of size.

Finally, hepatic resection for asymptomatic hepatic adenoma should be performed if malignant causes cannot be reasonably excluded. The inability to exclude malignant causes such as fibrolamellar hepatocellular carcinoma is a clear indication to offer resection to patients with asymptomatic hepatic adenomas.[16-18]

Adenoma rupture risk increases during pregnancy in an unpredictable manner and is associated with an increased risk of mortality to both mother and fetus. Thus, resection of hepatic adenomas prior to pregnancy is reasonable even if the patient is asymptomatic.[19-21] If hepatic adenomas are diagnosed during pregnancy, resection may be feasible, especially during the second trimester.[21] Hepatic adenomatosis patients with multiple adenomas, regardless of the absence of symptoms, are another at-risk group for bleeding and malignant transformation who should be offered hepatic resection.[22,23]

In contradistinction to the risk of inaction, the risk of elective hepatic resection is low with <1% mortality.[8] On the other hand, adenoma patients who are conservatively managed with observation face a 25% morbidity risk and a 5% to 20% mortality risk if emergent surgery is required for massive hemorrhagic rupture.[24,25]

Summary

The tipping point toward surgical resection in asymptomatic hepatic adenomas occurs when the risk of inaction and observation becomes greater than the risk of surgical resection. Given the risks of rupture, hemorrhage, and malignant transformation, the data—though limited—support resection when patients present with large (>5 cm) or multiple hepatic adenomas, especially if the lesions are peripheral. In the case of smaller lesions, resection should also be considered due to a persistent risk of malignant transformation.

KEY POINTS

- Complications of hepatic adenomas are common with an increased risk of rupture and bleeding.

- The risk of malignant transformation remains even with adenoma regression and oral contraceptive discontinuation.

- The risk of elective resection for hepatic adenomas is very low and far exceeded by the high risk if emergent surgery is required for hepatic adenoma complications.

COUNTERPOINT

Observe Asymptomatic Hepatic Adenomas

by Anjana Pillai, MD

Hepatic adenomas are uncommon, benign liver tumors classically seen in young women. The incidence has increased considerably due to their strong association with oral contraceptives (OCPs) and due to improved radiographic imaging leading to a rise in incidental findings.[26] Multiple studies have confirmed the relationship between the dose and duration of OCPs and the growth of hepatic adenomas.[26-28] Similarly, regression and/or resolution of adenomas have been demonstrated with the discontinuation of estrogen therapy.[12,29]

A fundamental feature separating hepatic adenomas from other benign tumors of the liver are their potential for spontaneous hemorrhage, rupture, and malignant transformation. As such, treatment strategies vary and a definitive solution to their management has yet to be established.

Historically, the management of asymptomatic hepatic adenomas was based on an arbitrary lesion size. Adenomas rarely have a fibrous capsule and can grow up to 30 cm.[30] As such, the majority were resected to avoid malignant transformation or hemorrhage.[11,30-32] However, the true risk of bleeding and malignant transformation of asymptomatic adenomas is unknown.

Until recently, only limited data were available on the outcomes of a conservative approach to adenoma patients. In a 2006 study of 48 female patients with hepatic adenomas, 58% were managed conservatively without surgical resection.[33] Median lesion size was 4 cm and ranged from 1 to 10 cm. During a 2-year follow-up, no lesion increased in size or had evidence of spontaneous hemorrhage or malignant transformation. In the group who underwent surgical resection to exclude malignancy, none of the lesions showed malignant transformation and 2 appeared to be primary hepatocellular carcinomas rather than adenomas. A more recent study examined both conservative and operative management of patients with benign hepatic tumors.[34] Seventy-five percent of the adenomas were <5 cm. All adenoma patients who were managed conservatively did well over a 6-year follow-up, with no evidence of spontaneous hemorrhage or malignant transformation, including 3 patients who had an increase in the size of their tumor. Similarly, in a study by Terkivatam et al, asymptomatic patients with adenomas <5 cm were observed over a mean follow-up period of 45 months and none had bleeding or malignant transformation.[31] Additionally, 43% of these adenomas regressed with cessation of OCPs.

As illustrated by the preceding studies, the overwhelming majority of patients with bleeding, spontaneous rupture, or malignant transformation were symptomatic and had large tumors, often >10 cm, and were rarely seen in tumors <5 cm.[10,31,33-37]

The risk of malignant transformation of adenomas has been reported to vary from 8% to 25%, but the data are based largely on case reports and retrospective studies with small cohorts of patients.[5,10,11,38,39] It is unclear from these studies if there was true malignant transformation or if this was an early presentation of hepatocellular carcinoma (HCC). In a 1994 review of the literature, only 5 clearly documented cases of HCC arising from an adenoma were found over a 30-year period.[10] In a Japanese study of benign hepatic lesions resected due to a preoperative diagnosis of malignancy, all adenomas were found to be free of malignant tumor upon excision.[40] In 2 other case reports of malignant transformation, patients were symptomatic (with 13 cm lesions) and 1 patient had marked elevations in her alpha-fetoprotein (AFP) level.[15,41] In a recent, single-center study of 122 patients with resected hepatic adenomas, 21% of patients had evidence of hemorrhage and 8% had malignant characteristics.[3] Of the 26 patients, 23 patients with hemorrhage were experiencing symptomatic abdominal pain and all had tumors >5 cm. HCC developed in large adenomas (>8 cm) in all cases except one. These studies suggest that smaller (<5 cm) adenomas are at significantly decreased risk of malignant transformation.

An additional argument against universal resection is the surgical risk. Despite marked advances in surgical techniques, the morbidity rate is as high as 25%, and the mortality rate remains near 1%.[35,36] The morbidity and mortality associated with surgery should be carefully explored given that the majority of these asymptomatic lesions are benign and there is a minimal risk of adverse outcomes.

Summary

Asymptomatic hepatic adenomas >5 cm can be considered for resection given the risk of bleeding, rupture, and malignant transformation. However, there are emerging data that warrant a shift in the treatment paradigm of smaller (<5 cm) adenomas. Given the fact that the vast majority of these smaller lesions will decrease in size or stabilize with the discontinuation of OCPs, and the fact that the risk of complications from these lesions appears minimal based on recent literature, a conservative approach with observation is warranted.

KEY POINTS

- Treatment strategies for asymptomatic adenomas are not well defined.
- Asymptomatic adenomas <5 cm can be observed safely.
- Larger adenomas can be considered for resection if they are enlarging or are symptomatic.
- Surgical risk has to be weighed carefully as mortality is near 1% and morbidity is as high as 25%.

Observation or Resection of Asymptomatic Hepatic Adenomas: A Summary and Recommendations

by Stanley Martin Cohen, MD

Excellent arguments are put forth by my colleagues on the approach to patients with hepatic adenomas. Dr. Pillai's position is that of observation based on the fact that complications occur in only a minority of cases and are almost nonexistent in adenomas <5 cm. She does concede, however, that adenomas >5 cm should likely be resected. But she brings up the point that resection of these lesions can be associated with significant surgical morbidity (up to 25%) and mortality (approximately 1%).

Dr. Ahn's position is that of resection of all asymptomatic adenomas because he believes that the complications are common enough and substantial enough to justify the surgical risks. He shows that the risk of rupture and bleeding (which increases with tumor size) is up to 25%, with a 20% mortality rate. He also comments on case reports of malignant transformation developing even after OCPs were stopped and the adenomas had radiographic regression or disappearance. He also notes that adenomas tend to occur in young women of child-bearing age and that the complication and morbidity/mortality rates may increase during pregnancy. He uses this as further evidence that all adenomas should be prophylactically resected. With regard to the surgical risks, he comments that the elective mortality rate of <1% is acceptable given the fact that the mortality rate can reach 25% if this surgery needs to be performed emergently.

The ultimate decision to resect or observe focuses on the risk of the adenoma causing complications versus the risk of surgical resection. Due to increased complication risks, several scenarios would probably be agreed upon by both of my colleagues as indications for resection. These would include large adenomas (>5 cm), symptomatic adenomas, adenomas with evidence of bleeding or impending rupture, hepatic adenomatosis (multiple adenomas), and any-sized adenomas in men.[3] Recent studies did not confirm a higher complication risk in pregnant women, and thus these patients should be treated similarly to a nonpregnant woman.[3,42]

The more controversial issue is the treatment of a woman with a solitary, smaller (<5 cm), asymptomatic adenoma. While uncommon, there have been reports of smaller adenomas bleeding and undergoing malignant transformation. This information would support an approach that all adenomas, regardless of size, should be resected. However, more recent studies have shown that smaller adenomas tend to remain stable or regress and have no associated complications during the follow-up period, supporting a conservative approach of just observing asymptomatic women with hepatic adenomas that are <5 cm.[3,34] These studies also showed major perioperative complication rates of 15% to 21% in those patients who did undergo resection.

Not addressed by my colleagues is the concept of determining the risk of complications based on the subtype of the adenoma. On MRI and/or biopsy, adenomas can be classified as steatotic, telangiectatic, or unclassified. The risk of complications from the steatotic adenomas is much lower than the other subtypes. The French study demonstrated that the telangiectatic subtype had the highest bleeding risk (30%).[3] Malignancy was found in 10% of the telangiectatic adenomas and 14% of the unclassified adenomas, but was not seen in the steatotic adenomas.

In the future, molecular markers such as β-catenin mutations (associated with a higher risk of malignant transformation) may provide further guidance in the decision of resection versus observation. Also, other treatment options including ablative therapies such as embolization and radiofrequency ablation may be proven to be effective curative therapies. Finally, laparoscopic surgical resection may be able to provide curative resection with lower morbidity and mortality than conventional surgical approaches.

Summary

Based on the information presented by my colleagues, I would favor a selective approach for the resection of asymptomatic adenomas:

1. All adenomas in men should be resected.

2. All adenomas >5 cm in women should be resected.

3. For adenomas <5 cm in women, the subtype of the adenoma should be determined either radiologically or pathologically to provide a risk assessment for adenma-related complications.

   - Telangiectatic—resection

   - Unclassified—resection

   - Steatotic—observe

4. Observed adenomas should be followed with imaging studies and resection should be considered if the lesions enlarge or if symptoms develop.

References

1. Colli A, Fraquelli M, Massironi S, et al. Elective surgery for benign liver tumors. *Cochrane Database Syst Rev.* 2007;24(1):CD005164.
2. Deneve JL, Pawlik TM, Cunningham S, et al. Liver cell adenoma: a multicenter analysis of risk factors for rupture and malignancy. *Ann Surg Oncol.* 2009;16:640-648.
3. Dokmak S, Paradis V, Vilgrain V, et al. A single-center surgical experience of 122 patients with single and multiple hepatocellular adenomas. *Gastroenterol.* 2009;137:1698-1705.
4. de Wilt JH, de Man RA, Lameris JS, et al. Hepatocellular adenoma in 20 patients: recommendations for treatment. *Ned Tijdschr Geneeskd.* 1998;142:2459-2463.
5. Leese T, Farges O, Bismuth H. Liver cell adenomas. A 12-year surgical experience from a specialist hepato-biliary unit. *Ann Surg.* 1988;208:558-564.
6. Cho SW, Marsh JW, Steel J, et al. Surgical management of hepatocellular adenoma: take it or leave it? *Ann Surg Oncol.* 2008;15:2795-2803.
7. Rubin RA, Mitchell DG. Evaluation of the solid hepatic mass. *Med Clin North Am.* 1996;80:907-928.
8. Shortell CK, Schwartz SI. Hepatic adenoma and focal nodular hyperplasia. *Surg Gynecol Obstet.* 1991;173:426-431.
9. Farges O, Dokmak S. Malignant transformation of liver adenoma: an analysis of the literature. *Dig Surg.* 2010;27:32-38.
10. Foster JH, Berman MM. The malignant transformation of liver cell adenomas. *Arch Surg.* 1994;129:712-717.
11. Ault GT, Wren SM, Ralls PW, et al. Selective management of hepatic adenomas. *Am Surg.* 1996;62:825-829.
12. Edmondson HA, Reynolds TB, Henderson B, et al. Regression of liver cell adenomas associated with oral contraceptives. *Ann Intern Med.* 1977;86:180-182.
13. Malt RA. Surgery for hepatic neoplasms. *N Engl J Med.* 1985;313:1591-1596.

14. Knowles DM, Casarella WJ, Johnson PM, et al. The clinical, radiologic, and pathologic characterization of benign hepatic neoplasms. Alleged association with oral contraceptives. *Medicine.* 1978;57:223-237.

15. Gyorffy EJ, Bredfeldt JE, Black WC. Transformation of hepatic cell adenoma to hepatocellular carcinoma due to oral contraceptive use. *Ann Intern Med.* 1989;110:489-490.

16. Choi BY, Nguyen MH. The diagnosis and management of benign hepatic tumors. *J Clin Gastro.* 2005;39:401-412.

17. Chen MF. Hepatic resection for benign tumors of the liver. *J Gastro Hep.* 2000;15:587-592.

18. Trotter JF, Everson GT. Benign focal lesions of the liver. *Clin Liv Dis.* 2001;5:17-42.

19. Monks PL, Fryar BG, Biggs WW. Spontaneous rupture of an hepatic adenoma in pregnancy with survival of mother and fetus. *Aust N Z J Obstet Gynaecol.* 1986;26:155-157.

20. Estebe JP, Malledant Y, Guillou YM, et al. Spontaneous rupture of an adenoma of the liver during pregnancy. *J Chir.* 1988;125:654-656.

21. Terkivatan, T, de Wilt, Jh, de Man, RA, et al. Management of hepatocellular adenoma during pregnancy. *Liver.* 2000;20:186-187.

22. Ribeiro A, Burgart LJ, Nagorney DM, et al. Management of liver adenomatosis: results with a conservative surgical approach. *Liver Transpl Surg.* 1998;4:388-398.

23. Grazioli L, Federle MP, Ichikawa T, et al. Liver adenomatosis: clinical, histopathologic, and imaging findings in 15 patients. *Radiology.* 2000;216:395-402.

24. Eckhauser FE, Knol JA, Raper SE, et al. Enucleation combined with hepatic vascular exclusion is a safe and effective alternative to hepatic resection for liver cell adenoma. *Am Surg.* 1994;60:466-471.

25. Chaib E, Gama-Rodrigues J, Ribeiro MA, et al. Hepatic adenoma. Timing for surgery. *Hepato-Gastroenterol.* 2007;54:1382-1387.

26. Baum JK, Bookstein JJ, Holtz F, et al. Possible association between benign hepatomas and oral contraceptives. *Lancet.* 1973;2:926-929.

27. Edmondson HA, Henderson B, Benton B. Liver-cell adenomas associated with the use of oral contraceptives. *N Engl J Med.* 1976;294:470-472.

28. Rooks JB, Ory HW, Ishak KG, et al. Epidemiology of hepatocellular adenoma. The role of contraceptive use. *JAMA.* 1979;242:644-648.

29. Aseni P, Sansalone CV, Sammartino C, et al. Rapid disappearance of hepatic adenoma after contraceptive withdrawal. *J Clin Gastroenterol.* 2001;33:234-236.

30. Choi BY, Nguyen MH. The diagnosis and management of benign hepatic tumors. *J Clin Gastroenterol.* 2005;39:401-412.

31. Terkivatam T, de Wilt JHW, de Man RA, et al. Indications and long-term outcome of treatment of benign hepatic tumors. *Arch Surg.* 2001;136:1033-1038.

32. Charny CK, Jarnagin WR, Schwartz LH, et al. Management of 155 patients with benign liver tumours. *Br J Surg.* 2001;88:808-813.

33. van der Windt DJ, Kok NFM, Hussain SM, et al. Case-oriented approach to the management of hepatocellular adenoma. *Br J Surg.* 2006;93:1495-1502.

34. Dardenne S, Hubert C, Sempoux C, et al. Conservative and operative management of benign solid hepatic tumours: a successful stratified algorithm. *Eur J Gastroenterol Hepatol.* 2010;22(11):1337-1344

35. Iwatsuki S, Todo S, Starzl T. Excisional therapy for benign hepatic lesions. *Surg Gynecol Obstet.* 1990;171:240-246.

36. Kammula US, Buell JF, Labow DM, et al. Surgical management of benign tumors of the liver. *Int J Gastrointest Cancer.* 2001;30:141-146.

37. Bahirwani R, Reddy KR. Review article: the evaluation of solitary liver masses. *Aliment Pharmacol Ther.* 2008;28:953-965.

38. Nagorney DM. Benign hepatic tumors: focal nodular hyperplasia and hepatocellular adenoma. *World J Surg.* 1995;19:13-18.

39. Kerlin P, Davis GL, McGill DB, et al. Hepatic adenoma and focal nodular hyperplasia: clinical, pathologic, and radiologic features. *Gastroenterol.* 1983;84:994-1002.

40. Shimizu S, Takayama T, Kosuge T, et al. Benign tumors of the liver resected because of a diagnosis of malignancy. *Surg Gynecol Obstet.* 1992;174:403-407.

41. Gordon SC, Reddy KR, Livingstone AS, et al. Resolution of a contraceptive-steroid-induced hepatic adenoma with subsequent evolution into hepatocellular carcinoma. *Ann Intern Med.* 1986;105:547-549.

42. Cobey FC, Salem RR. A review of liver masses in pregnancy and a proposed algorithm for their diagnosis and management. *Am J Surg.* 2004;187:181-191.

SECTION IV
OTHER CHRONIC LIVER DISEASES AND CIRRHOSIS

STRICTLY ADHERE TO THE "6-MONTH RULE" FOR RECENT HISTORY OF ALCOHOL ABUSE IN POTENTIAL LIVER TRANSPLANT CANDIDATES?

Parul Dureja Agarwal, MD and Michael Ronan Lucey, MD

Alcoholic liver disease (ALD) is the most common cause of cirrhosis in the Western world, and a leading indication for liver transplantation (LT). Starzl et al initially reported successful LT as treatment for patients with alcoholic liver disease (ALD).[1] Since then, many groups have reported successful transplants of patients with ALD, with alcoholic cirrhosis becoming one of the most common indications for LT. Several studies have reported that patient and graft survivals after LT for ALD are similar to or better than those for other indications.[2] Despite these advances, the majority of candidates with end-stage liver disease secondary to ALD in the United States who should be eligible for LT are not being referred to an LT center.

The present point/counterpoint will not address the biases that drive management of patients with alcoholic cirrhosis in the general community. Rather we will focus on a narrower controversy involving ALD patients who have found their way to an LT center: namely, the minimal duration of abstinence from alcohol (used synonymously with the term *sobriety* in this paper) that the LT center should require before admitting a candidate to the LT waiting list. As we shall see, the supporting data for any of the practical intervals are weak. Nonetheless, a 6-month abstinence period has been widely accepted in most centers in North America and Europe as a prerequisite for LT.[3]

The question therefore arises: how should transplant programs address recent alcohol use among alcoholic candidates for LT? It is now well recognized that 1- and 5-year patient and graft survivals after LT in selected patients with ALD are similar, if not better, than those for other indications.[4] Nevertheless, it is clear that up to 50% of alcoholic patients who receive a liver transplant will return to some drinking, and data are emerging that long-term survival may be impaired in alcoholic patients who return to addictive drinking.[5-7]

Jensen D.
Controversies in Hepatology: The Experts Analyze Both Sides (pp 103-110)
© 2011 SLACK Incorporated

In this argument and counterargument, we are concerned with patients with ALD who are in need of a LT, and whether a history of recent use of alcohol should influence selection and management. The scope of this challenge is shown by the fact that it is not limited to cirrhotic ALD patients with a recent decompensation due to alcohol use (alcohol-induced acute on chronic decompensation) but also includes patients with alcoholic hepatitis and cirrhotic ALD patients with HCC and recent alcohol use.

POINT

Transplant Programs Should Require 6 Months Abstinence When Selecting Liver Transplant Candidates With a History of Alcohol Dependence

by Parul Dureja Agarwal, MD

There are 3 broad explanations that might be used to justify the 6-month rule for abstinence prior to liver transplantation for ALD. These are that it is an important adjunct to treatment, or more specifically recovery, from liver failure; that it enables the transplant team to better predict future drinking; and that it is a punitive response to the behavior of the drinker. Let us consider each of these explanations in turn.

Recovery

One of the main putative advantages of the 6-month rule is that this period of pretransplant sobriety will allow the liver to recover, such that LT becomes unnecessary. It is beyond argument that continued alcohol consumption is detrimental to alcoholic cirrhotics and that stopping alcohol may allow recovery. This applies both in patients with alcoholic hepatitis and acute chronic decompensation.[8,9] Furthermore, a recent study regarding patients with moderately decompensated alcoholic cirrhosis (Child-Pugh class B) showed a survival benefit for standard medical care rather than proceeding to LT, indicating that a significant number of these patients show sufficient improvement with prolonged abstinence that they no longer need urgent LT.[10] The argument is, therefore, that forestalling transplantation for 6 months is necessary to allow spontaneous recovery to take place. However, controversy exists on setting the correct interval of time for observation and medical management. As we shall see in the following section, a strong case can be made for a 3-month interval.

Predicts Future Abstinence

Although data on alcohol relapse by alcoholics after LT leading to liver damage or graft loss are scanty, there is a clear consensus among transplant and addiction experts that alcoholic patients should abstain from alcohol after LT.[4] This is based on our understanding of the havoc wrecked on patients and families by alcohol dependency. Liver transplantation places great strain on patients and their families, and addictive drinking only exacerbates these strains.

Consequently, there is agreement that since alcoholism is a disorder of frequent relapse, an attempt to identify patients at greatest risk of relapse is appropriate.[11] It is against this background that the "6-month abstinence rule" has come into being. The choice of "6 months" is a compromise between wishing to have a longer period of abstinence and recognition of the acute urgency of many of these patients. Furthermore, although there are data on both sides of the issue, some studies have shown lower relapse rates among patients who were abstinent for 6 months or more.[12,13] Supported by these circumstances, most transplant centers in Europe and North America require an abstinence period of 6 months or more before placing an alcoholic patient on the transplant waiting list.[3]

Gives a Lower Priority to Patients With Alcoholic Liver Disease

This argument, articulated by Moss and Siegler, is based on the notion that alcoholics bear some responsibility for their plight, and therefore should be given lower priority than patients who have developed liver failure through (to use Moss and Siegler's phrase) "no fault of their own."[14] They further refine this by saying that the responsibility ignored by alcoholics is that of getting treatment for their condition.

KEY POINTS

- Six months provides an opportunity for alcoholic patients to recover from alcohol-induced decompensation or from alcoholic hepatitis.
- Six months may predict future abstinence, particularly after LT.
- To recognize that patients with ALD merit a lower priority for LT compared to nonalcoholic patients.

COUNTERPOINT

Transplant Programs Should Not Require 6 Months Abstinence When Selecting Liver Transplant Candidates With a History of Alcohol Dependence

by Michael Ronan Lucey, MD

Beginning with Starzl et al in 1988, many groups have reported successful transplants of patients with ALD, with alcoholic cirrhosis becoming one of the most common indications for liver transplantation in large data registries.[1] Several studies have reported that patient and graft survivals after OLT for ALD are comparable with those for other indications.[2,4] These advances have been made in the setting of selection practices aimed at identifying and excluding alcoholic patients considered to have the greatest risk of relapse into alcoholism after LT. The selection process is center specific but usually involves an assessment by an addiction professional, and in addition most commonly includes a required interval of reported abstinence from alcohol. In the United States, the requirement is often mandated by the payer. This counterargument will suggest that rigid adherence to a 6-month abstinence rule is a poor way to identify patients likely to relapse and is punitive to some others who will not.

Recovery

Six months is an arbitrary threshold for abstinence, which is open to challenge. Veldt et al published a retrospective analysis of alcoholic patients admitted to the hospital with decompensation precipitated by recent alcohol use and showed that no further improvement in liver function occurred after 3 months of abstinence.[15] Thus, while a pre-LT abstinence period gives an opportunity to those patients who will recover their liver function, the arbitrary choice of 6 months puts some abstinent patients in jeopardy of dying during the interval of abstinence.

Predicts Future Abstinence

Although 6 months of abstinence is a widely accepted standard, it is important to acknowledge its limitations. First, most studies of alcohol relapse after LT are retrospective and based on selection practices that included the 6-month abstinence rule. Indeed, the failure to prevent alcohol use in these studies is more an indictment of the 6-month rule rather than a confirmation of its efficacy.

That is not to say that duration of abstinence has no value. It has been shown in both retrospective and prospective studies that the greater the interval of abstinence the more likely the subject would maintain abstinence after LT, though 6 months abstinence of itself is of little value.[2,16] These studies are similarly confounded by the use of the 6-month rule in the selection process.

Second, the emphasis on the dichotomy of abstinence/drinking, while appropriate in advising patients, is naïve in relation to the nature of alcoholism and addiction. Alcohol dependence is a chronic disorder in which relapse is very common. As such, the observation that approximately 50% of alcoholic LT recipients admit to some alcohol use and 10% to 15% acknowledge abusive drinking needs to be carefully parsed. There are several patterns of alcohol relapse, from the one-time slip to the resumption of frequent excessive use, with many variants in between. Unfortunately, we have very little data on better methods of screening for patients with the greater risk of returning to the most injurious patterns of drinking. This has not been assessed in relation to the 6-month rule.

Third, it is necessary to consider those patients who will die without LT as a result of strict adherence to the 6-month abstinence rule, since it is probable that some of them would not have relapsed to alcohol use after LT, or, at least, would not have succumbed to alcoholic damage to the allograft. Patients with severe alcoholic hepatitis (AH) are a particular subgroup of alcoholic patients in this respect, since they have been excluded from most considerations of treatment with LT.[17] As a consequence of the 6-month rule, many patients with the severest form of AH, who have failed to improve with medical management with prednisolone, have not been offered LT, despite having a very high short-term mortality. At the 2009 American Association for the Study of Liver Diseases Liver Meeting, Mathurin et al[18] presented preliminary data drawn from a prospective study with historical case controls of early LT applied to carefully-selected patients with severe AH who had failed to respond to prednisolone. Patient survival at 6 months in the first 18 subjects was 83.3% amongst the transplanted group, compared to 44.4% in the control group. Further, there was no relapse to alcohol use in the first year amongst the early transplanted group. We await the completion of this study, which seems likely to challenge the dominant viewpoint that LT is not an appropriate therapy in patients with AH, irrespective of their psychosocial assessment or level of urgency.

Give a Lower Priority to Patients With Alcoholic Liver Disease

It should be stated that Moss and Siegler's justification of their proposed policy to limit access of alcoholics to LT did not include consideration of the 6-month rule.[14] Similarly, subsequent writers on the 6-month rule have not sought to justify the rule as a punitive response to alcoholism. Lastly, Benjamin and Turcotte have provided a comprehensive rebuttal of Moss and Siegler, arguing that their polemic lacked foundation in understanding alcoholism or addiction, that Moss and Siegler's emphasis on the responsibility of the alcoholic to seek treatment was undermined by the disappointing efficacy of treatment for alcoholism, and that similar considerations were not applied to other disorders of the liver wherein volition played a part in the development of liver injury.[19] Hepatitis C and B infection and nonalcoholic steatohepatitis as part of the metabolic syndrome would often fall into this category.

KEY POINTS

- Six months is excessive as an interval to discover which patients will recover from alcohol-induced decompensation or from alcoholic hepatitis. This will be apparent after 3 months. Salvageable patients will die in the second 3 months.

- Six months abstinence is a poor predictor of abstinence after LT. While all prediction is flawed, a comprehensive assessment by an addiction specialist is better than the 6-month rule.

- Few authorities accept that patients with ALD merit a lower priority for LT compared to nonalcoholic patients.

EXPERT OPINION

Universally Accepted, But Should Not Be a Barrier for Transplantation

by Parul Dureja Agarwal, MD and Michael Ronan Lucey, MD

Notwithstanding multiple studies in this area, no predefined duration of pretransplant abstinence has emerged that can reliably be used as a "cutoff" to predict those likely to relapse to alcohol use post-LT, while not denying suitable patient access. Nonetheless, a 6-month abstinence period has been widely accepted in most centers in North America and Europe as a prerequisite for liver transplantation. We believe that a balanced reading of the available data indicates that 6 months abstinence is of little prognostic value when used as a sole criterion for predicting future alcohol use. Sobriety of less than 6 months duration should not, on its own, constitute a barrier to liver transplantation in an otherwise suitable candidate. We advocate for evaluation by a skilled addiction professional that considers other prognostic factors such as the understanding of addiction by the patient; his or her previous history with regard to abstinence and treatment; his or her interest in and willingness to undergo treatment where appropriate; the presence of psychiatric comorbidities including active polysubstance abuse; and the stability of his or her relationships, housing and employment.[11] A comprehensive evaluation that considers the whole patient is a better way to assess the patient's risk of relapse.

References

1. Starzl TE, Van Thiel D, Tzakis AG, et al. Orthotopic liver transplantation for alcoholic cirrhosis. *JAMA.* 1988;260:2542-2544.
2. Lucey MR, Schaubel DE, Guidinger MK, et al. Effects of alcoholic liver disease and hepatitis C infection on waiting list and posttransplant mortality and transplant survival benefit. *Hepatology.* 2009;50:400-406.
3. Everhart JE, Beresford TP . Liver transplantation for alcoholic liver disease: a survey of transplantation programs in the United States. *Liver Transpl Surg.* 1997;3:220-226.
4. Weinrieb RM, Lucey MR. Liver Transplantation for Alcoholic Liver Disease. In: Busuttil RW, Klintmalm GB, eds. *For Transplantation of the Liver, Second Edition.* New York, NY: Elsevier Science; 2005.
5. DiMartini A, Day N, Dew MA, et al. Alcohol consumption patterns and predictors of use following liver transplantation for alcoholic liver disease. *Liver Transpl.* 2006;12:813-820.
6. Cuadrado A, Fabrega E, Casafont F, et al. Alcoholic recidivism impairs long tern patient survival after orthotopic liver transplantation for alcoholic liver disease. *Liver Transpl.* 2005;11:420-426.
7. Pfitzmann R, Schwenzer J, Rayes N, et al. Long-term survival and predictors of relapse after orthotopic liver transplantation for alcoholic liver disease. *Liver Transpl.* 2007;13:197-205.
8. Powell WJ Jr, Klatskin G. Duration of survival in patients with Laennec's cirrhosis: Influence of alcohol withdrawal, and possible effects of recent changes in general management of the disease. *Am J Med.* 1968;44:406-420.
9. Alexander JF, Lischner MW, Galambos JT. Natural history of alcoholic hepatitis II. *Am J. Gastroenterol.* 1971;56:515-525.
10. Vanlemmnes C, Di Martino V, Milan C, et al. Immediate listing for liver transplantation versus standard care for Child-Pugh B alcoholic cirrhosis: a randomized trial. *Ann Intern Med.* 2009;150:153-161.
11. Beresford TP. The psychiatric evaluation of the liver transplant candidate with alcoholic cirrhosis. In: Lucey MR, Merion RM, Beresford TP, eds. *Liver Transplantation and the Alcoholic Patient.* Cambridge: Cambridge University Press; 1994.
12. Osorio RW, Ascher NL, Avery M, et al. Predicting recidivism after orthotopic liver transplantation for alcoholic liver disease. *Hepatology.* 1994;20:105-110.
13. Karim Z, Pongphob I, Scudamore CH, et al. Predictors of relapse to significant alcohol drinking after liver transplantation. *Can J Gastroenterol.* 2010;24:245-250.
14. Moss AH, Siegler M. Should alcoholics compete equally for liver transplantation? *JAMA.* 1991;265:1295-1298.
15. Veldt BJ, Laine F, Guillygomarc'h A, et al. Indication of liver transplantation in severe alcoholic liver cirrhosis: qualitative evaluation and optimal timing. *J Hepatol.* 2002;36:93.
16. Lucey MR, Merion RM, Henley KS, et al. Selection for and outcome of liver transplantation in alcoholic liver disease. *Gastroenterology.* 1992;102:1736-1741.

17. Lucey MR, Brown KA, Everson GT, et al. Minimal criteria for placement of adults on the liver transplant waiting list: a report of a national conference organized by the American Society of Transplant Physicians and the American Association for the Study of Liver Diseases. *Liver Transpl Surg.* 1997;3:628-637.
18. Mathurin P, Moreno C, Samuel D, et al. Early liver transplantation: a rescue option for patients with severe alcoholic hepatitis non-responsive to therapy. Presented at the American Association for the Study of Liver Diseases Liver Meeting; 2009.
19. Benjamin M, Turcotte J. Ethics of liver transplantaiton in the alcoholic patients. In: Lucey MR, Merion RM, Beresford TP, eds. *Liver Transplantation and the Alcoholic Patient.* Cambridge: Cambridge University Press, 1994.

CHAPTER 12

SHOULD LIVER BIOPSY BE PERFORMED IN ALL PATIENTS WITH NONALCOHOLIC FATTY LIVER DISEASE?

Neehar D. Parikh, MD; Lisa VanWagner, MD; and Mary E. Rinella, MD

Nonalcoholic fatty liver disease (NAFLD) is the most common cause of abnormal liver tests and a rising indication for liver transplantation. Nonalcoholic steatohepatitis (NASH), under the umbrella of NAFLD, has a more progressive course that results in cirrhosis in up to 20% of cases. It is such patients that need to be identified for directed therapeutic intervention in an attempt to reverse or, at minimum, stabilize liver injury.

POINT

Liver Biopsy Should Be Performed in All Patients With Nonalcoholic Fatty Liver Disease

by Neehar D. Parikh, MD

With the mounting obesity epidemic, the prevalence of NAFLD has increased to a projected 30% of the US population. Naturally, clinicians are frequently faced with how to best evaluate the patient suspected of having NAFLD. Once other causes are excluded serologically, liver biopsy is traditionally the next step in the diagnostic algorithm and the current state of the art supports this strategy.

Jensen D.
Controversies in Hepatology: The Experts Analyze Both Sides (pp 111-122)
© 2011 SLACK Incorporated

The prevalence of NAFLD in the Western world is approximated to be 20% to 30% of the general population and its most progressive form, nonalcoholic steatohepatitis (NASH)-induced cirrhosis, promises to be an ever increasing indication for liver transplantation. The histologic spectrum of NAFLD can be divided into "simple" steatosis and NASH, which, by definition, also includes evidence of cellular injury (ballooning change) and may include features such as steatonecrosis or fibrosis in the setting of hepatic steatosis.[1,2] This distinction is important due to differences in management and patient prognosis. While patients with "simple" steatosis rarely progress to cirrhosis (up to 3%), up to 20% of patients with NASH progress to cirrhosis. Furthermore, patients with NAFLD have a higher mortality than the general population, and this difference becomes more pronounced in those with NASH.[3]

Even the diagnosis of hepatic steatosis alone can help motivate patients and draw attention to related comorbidities that may otherwise not have been appreciated such as insulin resistance, dyslipidemia, and obstructive sleep apnea.[4] The most common cause of death in patients with NAFLD is cardiovascular disease and may play a role in atherosclerosis, endothelial function, and cardiac ATP reserve.[5-7] Several studies have now demonstrated that hepatic steatosis may be an independent risk factor for cardiovascular disease.[8-11] Thus, definitive diagnosis of NAFLD or NASH may assist clinicians in primary prevention of cardiovascular disease.

Serological Testing Is Neither Sensitive Nor Specific in Nonalcoholic Fatty Liver Disease

Noninvasive testing for the presence of fatty liver relies on a combination of laboratory tests and imaging. The central questions are whether noninvasive testing is a reliable proxy in NAFLD to distinguish simple steatosis from NASH and to detect and quantify hepatic fibrosis. Clinicians rely on abnormalities in liver chemistry tests to suggest the presence of NAFLD.[12] However, these laboratory tests have significant limitations, especially when interpreted in isolation. For example, in a study of 458 patients with NAFLD, 59% of patients with a normal ALT were found to have NASH on liver biopsy.[12] Alternatively, many investigators have attempted to derive scoring systems for NAFLD based upon laboratory tests and patient characteristics (eg, age and body mass index [BMI]). Examples include the BAAT score (BMI, ALT, age, and triglycerides),[13] FibroTest/FibroSure score (BioPredictive, Paris, France),[14] NAFLD fibrosis score,[15] BARD score (BMI ≥28 = 1 point, AAR of ≥0.8 = 2 points, DM = 1 point),[16] European liver fibrosis panel,[17] and FibroMeter (BD Diagnositc Systems, Sparks, MD).[18] While these composite tests can be effective in detecting NAFLD, their routine use is limited by suboptimal sensitivity and specificity in distinguishing those patients with NASH and/or early hepatic fibrosis from those with less advanced disease.[19,20]

Imaging Techniques Are Unable to Assess Disease Activity or Severity

Current imaging modalities are limited in their diagnostic capabilities. Ultrasound is highly sensitive for the detection of steatosis greater than 30%, and while CT and MRI are able to detect lesser degrees of steatosis, none of these modalities can distinguish NASH from simple steatosis.[21] Many strategies are emerging to quantify hepatic fibrosis. One of these is transient elastography (Fibroscan), a device designed to measure liver stiffness via pulse ultrasonography, which is not currently available for routine use in the United States.[22] In a cohort of 309 patients with NAFLD, compared with biopsy, transient elastography had a sensitivity and specificity of approximately 90% in cases of advanced fibrosis and cirrhosis; the specificity, however, was reduced to 50% in cases of mild fibrosis.[23] Importantly, transient elastography is limited in obese patients. Foucher et al reported a BMI >28 was associated with a failed test (odds ratio 10.0; 95% confidence interval, 5.7 to 17.9; $P = 0.0001$),[24] which is a major limitation in the NAFLD patient population.

The identification of early cirrhosis or advanced stage fibrosis allows surveillance for esophageal varices and hepatocellular carcinoma, both of which have available treatment modalities. As newer technologies are developed and validated (ie, MR elastography), the role of imaging for the noninvasive detection of early to moderate degrees of fibrosis may change. However, the current state of the art is not sufficiently reliable to supplant liver biopsy to stage fibrosis.

It Is Essential to Distinguish Nonalcoholic Steatohepatitis From Simple Steatosis

Distinguishing NASH from simple steatosis is relevant with respect to prognosis and the management of patients. Compared to the general NAFLD population, patients with NASH have higher liver-related and cardiovascular mortality.[6,25] Up until recently, no randomized controlled trial of sufficient size had been published to guide the therapy of patients with NASH. Recently, Sanyal et al found that compared to placebo, both vitamin E and pioglitazone improved liver enzymes, steatosis, and lobular inflammation, and, additionally, vitamin E improved NASH severity on biopsy in nondiabetic patients with NASH.[26] Furthermore, the benefits of surgical or non-surgical weight loss have been demonstrated in several publications.[27,28] These data show that the natural history of NAFLD and NASH can be altered by treatment interventions.

Summary

While there is small risk associated with liver biopsy,[29] noninvasive modalities are not accurate enough to provide the necessary clinical information to appropriately treat patients with NAFLD. No noninvasive test has been validated as an accurate and reliable method to distinguish NAFLD from NASH, determine grade severity, and determine the degree of fibrosis. Although some imaging modalities are fairly accurate at diagnosing cirrhosis, we remain without a reliable method to diagnose mild to moderate degrees of fibrosis, which may be reversible. These limitations are clinically relevant because at this time, noninvasive testing is unable to provide the key information to determine prognosis and determine eligibility for therapeutic interventions, whereas biopsy provides this information. Emerging therapies for NASH, especially pioglitazone, should only be given to patients with a biopsy-proven diagnosis due to risks associated with its use (heart failure, bone loss, and weight gain).[26] Thus, until noninvasive measures are available to reliably predict NASH and grade disease severity, the benefit of information obtained from liver biopsy will continue to outweigh potential risks.

KEY POINTS

- Serological tests have poor sensitivity and specificity in detecting NASH.
- Current imaging techniques are unable to distinguish patients with NASH.
- Detecting NASH and cirrhosis have important implications on management and prognosis.
- No noninvasive testing is sufficiently accurate, disseminated, or validated for widespread use.

COUNTERPOINT

Liver Biopsy Should Not Be Performed in All Patients With Nonalcoholic Fatty Liver Disease

by Lisa VanWagner, MD

In order to diagnose NASH with precision and characterize its severity, many argue that there is no substitute for performing a liver biopsy. A liver biopsy provides important information regarding the degree of liver damage, changes in the overall liver architecture, and the severity of inflammatory activity and fibrosis.[30,31] Although it is considered by many to be the gold standard for diagnosis, it is an imperfect standard that has many drawbacks. Thus, there are several significant limitations to proceeding with liver biopsy in all patients thought to have NAFLD.

First, there is an evolving consensus on a precise pathological definition of NASH and a system to grade its severity. The initial descriptions define NASH as the association of a fatty liver with inflammation, regardless of the presence of associated liver abnormalities.[32] Later, it was suggested that a fatty liver with inflammation alone (steatohepatitis) was not specific and that some degree of liver cell death (steatonecrosis) was required to diagnose NASH.[33] Current research criteria acknowledges the importance of fatty infiltration, inflammation, and cell death, but the variation in scoring systems used throughout research studies makes comparison of outcomes very difficult.[34] In addition, there is significant variability in histopathologic interpretations between even experienced pathologists. Several studies have demonstrated good inter-observer and intra-observer agreement in evaluation of the extent of steatosis and grade of fibrosis, but poor reliability in terms of cellular ballooning and lobular inflammation, which are key components for an accurate diagnosis of NASH.[35-37] In addition, diagnostic errors made by community pathologists have been reported in more than 25% of patients undergoing evaluation at academic centers.[38]

In addition to variability in pathologic interpretation, liver biopsy is subject to sampling error, which is in large part due to inconsistency in specimen size and the number of scores obtained.[30,37] Experts have also not reached agreement over the number of complete portal tracts required to make an accurate diagnosis.[39] Other important factors such as biopsy method (percutaneous, transjugular, or surgical) and timing of specimen acquisition during surgery can alter the interpretation of liver biopsy specimens, particularly with respect to fibrosis and inflammation, which are both important to determine the diagnosis of NASH and degree of liver injury.[31] Furthermore, differences can be seen between paired biopsies taken from the same lobe or different lobes of the same patient.[30,37,40,41]

Complications and Cost of Liver Biopsy Limit Its Broad Use

Liver biopsy is an invasive procedure with rare but potentially lethal complications. The overall mortality rate for percutaneous liver biopsy is as high as 1 in 10,000.[42] In general, the most common complaints after liver biopsy are pain, localized bleeding, and hypotension, which is the most common indication for hospitalization following liver biopsy.[43] At the Mayo Clinic, where most liver biopsies are done on outpatients, the risk for hospitalization after liver biopsy is estimated to be as high as 5%.[44] Although pain is dismissed as a trivial complication, it is experienced in 84% of individuals during liver biopsy, is "severe" in 20%, and may persist beyond the day of procedure.[45] Other rare complications of percutaneous liver biopsy include transient bacteremia, biliary ascites, bile pleuritis, bile peritonitis, pneumothorax, hemothorax, subcutaneous emphysema, pneumoperitoneum, pneumoscrotum, subphrenic abscess, pancreatitis due to hemobilia, and breakage of the biopsy needle.[39] With transjugular liver biopsy, the liver tissue is obtained from within the vascular system, which minimizes the risk of bleeding. However, complications associated with transjugular liver biopsy range from 1.3% to 20.2%, and mortality ranges from 0.1% to 0.5%.[46] Complications of transjugular liver biopsy include abdominal pain, neck hematoma, transient Horner syndrome, transient dysphonia, cardiac arrhythmias, pneumothorax, formation of a fistula from the hepatic artery to the portal vein or the biliary tree, perforation of the liver capsule (especially in small, cirrhotic livers), and death.[46] One must acknowledge, however, that patients undergoing transjugular biopsy are usually sicker and at higher risk for complications. Finally, because of the monitoring, processing, and interpretation required, the cost of liver biopsy is significant. A liver biopsy at most hospitals in the United States costs approximately $2200.[47] This cost does not include the additional expenses of hospitalization and treatment for patients who develop complications from the procedure or lost revenue.

Noninvasive Markers as an Alternative to Liver Biopsy

In light of the cost and invasive nature of liver biopsy, several noninvasive diagnostic tests have been developed. Examples include the FibroTest/FibroSure or FibroSpect (Prometheus Laboratories Inc., San Diego, CA) which estimate liver fibrosis[48] and SteatoTest, which estimates steatosis.[14] These and other proprietary panels have been extensively studied in chronic hepatitis C and more recently in NASH and combine various biochemical markers to predict disease stage. In addition to these composite tests, numerous circulating biomarkers and prediction models have been investigated to noninvasively predict hepatic histology in patients with NAFLD, although the full discussion is beyond the scope of this argument.[49] However, one promising biomarker, cytokeratin 18 (CK-18), has been consistently shown to be elevated in patients with NASH.[50-52] The rationale behind the use of CK-18 as a potential biomarker of disease activity is evidence that hepatocyte apoptosis may play an important role in the pathogenesis of NAFLD.[52] CK-18 is a major intermediate filament protein in hepatocytes that is cleaved by the effector caspases (mainly caspase 3) upon the activation of the apoptosis cascade.[53] Compared to individuals with normal histology and those without NASH, patients with definite NASH have significantly higher CK-18 fragment levels.[52] In addition to chemical biomarkers, noninvasive imaging techniques such as several magnetic resonance imaging (MRI)-based techniques including chemical shift imaging, frequency-selective imaging, MR elastography, and MR spectroscopy have been evaluated for use in detecting and quantifying liver steatosis and fibrosis and assessing inflammatory activity with promising results.[54,55] Studies of patients with chronic liver disease of various causes and varying degrees of severity have shown a good correlation ($r = 0.7$ to 0.99) between MR spectroscopy liver fat quantification and biochemical and histopathologic analyses.[54,55] The advantages offered by MR spectroscopy for fat quantification are its ability to determine the absolute liver fat concentration and its high sensitivity for detecting small amounts of hepatic triglyceride and subtle changes in hepatic triglyceride content during treatment. It is also useful for revealing a necroinflammatory response in the setting of chronic liver disease.[56] In addition to liver fat quantification and concentration, MR-based techniques are able to predict the degree of liver fibrosis, which may identify patients at risk for progressing to cirrhosis over time.

Liver Biopsy Findings Do Not Alter Management

Despite the limitations of noninvasive techniques to date, a liver biopsy often does not change management in a patient suspected to have NAFLD. Weight loss and treatment of comorbidities such as diabetes, hypertension, and hyperlipidemia have a beneficial effect on NAFLD and NASH.[57] In a pilot study, Ueno et al[57,58] examined the effects of a restricted diet and exercise regimen (walking or jogging) in obese Japanese subjects. After 3 months, the treated group had significant improvements in aminotransferases, total cholesterol, fasting glucose, BMI, and steatosis compared to the controls.[57,58] These interventions are noninvasive with few associated side effects, and thus, on a practical level, biopsy results are not generally needed to make these conservative recommendations. Furthermore, the largest randomized controlled trial in non-diabetic patients with NASH recently demonstrated that vitamin E effectively reduced NASH histological activity and improved liver enzymes. Despite the potential cardiac side effects associated with vitamin E, the risk is not prohibitive to preclude treatment without a liver biopsy proven diagnosis of NASH.[26,59]

Summary

Although liver biopsy is often considered to be the gold standard for the diagnosis of NAFLD or NASH, it is an imperfect standard. Liver biopsy is an expensive, invasive procedure with potentially serious complications that has limited accuracy due to sampling variability and histopathologic interpretation. Overall, liver biopsy often does little to change pre-test probability of NAFLD diagnosis, and treatment options are currently limited for early NAFLD and even NASH. Performing liver biopsies on 80 million Americans thought to have risk factors for NAFLD is not a reasonable option. Therefore, given the high prevalence of NAFLD and lack of pharmacological treatments available, it makes more sense to rely on clinical parameters, imaging, and available biomarkers.

KEY POINTS

- Lack of concensus regarding histologic diagnostic criteria for NASH.
- Variability in histopathologic interpretation between even expert pathologists.
- Liver biopsy is costly and impractical to perform in 80 million Americans.
- Noninvasive biomarkers and imaging studies appear promising.
- Liver biopsy may not change post-test probability of disease presence.

EXPERT OPINION

Liver Biopsy Still Plays an Important Role in the Diagnosis and Management of Nonalcoholic Steatohepatitis

by Mary E. Rinella, MD

Like all worthy controversies, valid arguments can be made on both sides of the question, and in this author's opinion, liver biopsy continues to provide useful information relevant to the diagnosis and treatment of NASH. Liver biopsy is still considered the "gold standard" for the diagnosis of NASH; however, it has many limitations, including sampling error, inter-observer variability in interpretation, and risk. An estimated 100 million people in the United States have NAFLD and liver biopsy is not necessary, practical, or appropriate in all patients with presumed NAFLD. Rather, as a clinician, the decision of whom to biopsy should be dictated by how one plans to use the biopsy results. With careful patient selection, liver biopsy can provide invaluable information. Liver biopsy can be utilized to diagnose NAFLD, distinguish NASH within the context of NAFLD and determine disease severity. It can also exclude other causes of liver disease in a patient with suspected NAFLD, and identify patients that may benefit from therapy.

Liver Biopsy to Determine the Presence of Nonalcoholic Fatty Liver Disease

NAFLD is the most common cause of abnormal liver chemistry tests and the most common reason for referral to a hepatologist. While simple steatosis has less liver-related morbidity and mortality than NASH, it is not entirely benign, with 4% developing cirrhosis and 2% developing liver-related mortality over an 8-year period.[32] Importantly, as described above, NAFLD is also associated with cardiovascular and other metabolic comorbidities. Inexpensive radiologic imaging, such as ultrasound, is able to detect the presence of significant steatosis. However, in patients who have less than 30% steatosis in the liver, diagnosis by ultrasound is less reliable. An important thing to note is that ultrasound is often unable to distinguish fat from fibrosis and this needs to be taken into consideration when interpreting results. More costly tests such as MRI can detect as little as 5% steatosis in the liver.[60] In the majority of cases, a presumptive diagnosis of NAFLD can be made and potentially corroborated by improvement in liver chemistry tests and reduction in the steatosis by imaging after weight loss without the need for liver biopsy. However, the answer to the more pertinent question, "Does the patient have NASH?" is not as straightforward.

Liver Biopsy to Distinguish Nonalcoholic Steatohepatitis From Simple Steatosis and Assess Disease Severity

Despite the emergence of promising biomarkers, liver biopsy with its known limitations remains the only reliable and accurate way to distinguish NASH from simple steatosis. Surrogate markers for hepatic inflammation and injury, including aminotransferases in the setting of NASH, remained limited, although more comprehensive diagnostic panels are being evaluated.[61] Noninvasive modalities have predominantly focused on the diagnosis of advanced fibrosis. However, many would argue that surrogate markers of inflammation and injury are more pertinent to NASH.[15-17,62-65]

Although over 100 papers have been published over the last 10 years evaluating potential biomarkers for NASH, we remain without a reliable, accurate, readily available biomarker to distinguish NASH from simple hepatic steatosis. In contrast to other forms of liver disease, liver enzymes are not reliably elevated in patients with NASH. In fact, one study determined that abnormal liver enzymes had a positive predictive value of only 34% for the diagnosis of NASH. Furthermore, patients with advanced steatohepatitis, including cirrhosis, can have normal liver enzymes and—in many patients—the degree of hepatic steatosis will decrease as NASH becomes more progressive.[66] Biomarkers of inflammation such as TNF-α and IL-6 and markers of oxidative stress including byproducts of lipid peroxidation have been shown to correlate with steatohepatitis. To date, the most promising biomarker is cytokeratin 18, which is a byproduct of apoptosis.[23] Elevated levels of CK-18 have a positive and negative predictive value for the diagnosis of NASH of 99.9% and 85.7%, respectively.[52,67] This has recently been validated in a multicenter study with a diverse NASH population as an independent predictor of NASH with an area under the receiver operating characteristic (ROC) curve (AUC) of 0.83.[68]

Clinical predictors such as BMI or waist circumference, the presence of severe insulin resistance or diabetes, hypertension, and race used independently or within the context of a predictive model are helpful in assessing the relative probability that a patient with hepatic steatosis has NASH. Although very helpful, these surrogate markers do not offer a high enough sensitivity and specificity to supplant liver biopsy at this time. Furthermore, knowing the extent of liver injury also offers prognostic information and helps identify patients with early cirrhosis that might benefit from screening for hepatocellular carcinoma or esophageal varices.

Serum fibrosis markers have also been extensively studied and are fairly effective for the diagnosis of advanced fibrosis. A study validating the Enhanced Liver Fibrosis (ELF) panel—a predictive model derived from hyaluronic acid, aminoterminal peptide of protocollagen 3 (PIIINP) and tissue inhibitor of matrix metallic proteinase-1 (TIMP-1)—in 196 patients with NAFLD had an AUC of 0.9 to detect advanced fibrosis. In this cohort only 14% of patients would have had an indeterminate score that prompted liver biopsy. Overall, this and other methods including radiologic methods are fairly reliable to diagnose advanced fibrosis or cirrhosis, although they lack accuracy in lesser or more moderate degrees of fibrosis. Therefore, to assess the degree of fibrosis in a patient with NASH, it may be appropriate to use noninvasive modalities and limit liver biopsy to those with indeterminate values.

Liver Biopsy to Exclude Other Liver Diseases

Some patients with suspected NAFLD have other causes of liver injury in addition to or in lieu of NAFLD. Therefore, alternative explanations for abnormal liver chemistry tests need to be sought and excluded: excessive alcohol use, viral hepatitis, Wilson's disease, and autoimmune liver disease, among others. In up to 33% of patients, autoimmune markers such as antinuclear antibody and antismooth muscle antibody are positive in patients with NAFLD and a liver biopsy is useful to exclude the presence of autoimmune hepatitis. Although in one study, 66% of 354 patients with a negative serological evaluation had NAFLD or NASH, the remainder had other diseases diagnosed on biopsy such as drug-induced liver injury, autoimmune liver disease, or cryptogenic hepatitis.[69]

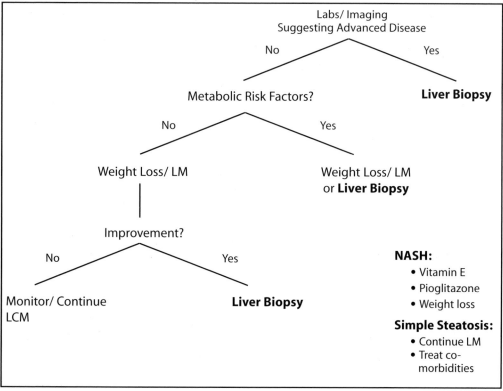

Figure 12-1. Proposed algorithm for liver biopsy in a patient with negative serological evaluation and suspected NAFLD. LM= lifestyle modification.

Liver Biopsy to Guide Management in Patients With NASH

Establishing a diagnosis of steatohepatitis and documenting the degree of liver injury and fibrosis is very important (Figure 12-1). Up until recently, one could argue that no effective treatments were available, making justification for liver biopsy in NASH more contentious. Vitamin E is effective and fairly safe, although cardiovascular and bleeding issues have been raised. Pioglitazone is effective in improving some histologic features of NASH and has the additional benefit of decreasing insulin resistance; however, it is associated with potentially serious adverse effects.[26] For many patients, bariatric surgery is the only way to achieve and maintain weight loss. Bariatric surgery can be quite effective in such patients and has been shown to improve NASH in addition to its other established benefits. While offering a treatment with a low side effect empirically may be appropriate, more high risk or invasive interventions should be justified only by the presence of more advanced disease. Therefore, a liver biopsy demonstrating moderate to severe NASH can guide the use of interventions such as pioglitazone or bariatric surgery.

References

1. Chalasani N, Wilson L, Kleiner DE, et al. Relationship of steatosis grade and zonal location to his-tological features of steatohepatitis in adult patients with non-alcoholic fatty liver disease. *J Hepatol.* 2008;48(5):829-834.

2. Matteoni CA, Younossi ZM, Gramlich T, et al. Nonalcoholic fatty liver disease: a spectrum of clinical and pathological severity. *Gastroenterol.* 1999;116(6):1413-1419.

3. Soderberg C, Stal P, Askling J, et al. Decreased survival of subjects with elevated liver function tests during a 28-year follow-up. *Hepatology.* 2010;51(2):595-602.

4. Mishra P, Nugent C, Afendy A, et al. Apnoeic-hypopnoeic episodes during obstructive sleep apnoea are associated with histological nonalcoholic steatohepatitis. *Liver Int.* 2008;28(8):1080-1086.

5. Adams LA, Lymp JF, St Sauver J, et al. The natural history of nonalcoholic fatty liver disease: a popu-lation-based cohort study. *Gastroenterology.* 2005;129(1):113-121.

6. Söderberg C, Stål P, Askling J, et al. Decreased survival of subjects with elevated liver function tests during a 28-year follow-up. *Hepatology.* 2010;51(2):595-602.

7. Sookoian S, Pirola CJ. Non-alcoholic fatty liver disease is strongly associated with carotid atheroscle-rosis: a systematic review. *J Hepatol.* 2008;49(4):600-607.

8. Caserta CA, Pendino GM, Amante A, et al. Cardiovascular risk factors, nonalcoholic fatty liver disease, and carotid artery intima-media thickness in an adolescent population in southern Italy. *Am J Epidemiol.* 2010;171(11):1195-1202.

9. Targher G, Bertolini L, Padovani R, et al. Relations between carotid artery wall thickness and liver histology in subjects with nonalcoholic fatty liver disease. *Diabetes Care.* 2006;29(6):1325-1330.

10. Targher G, Bertolini L, Poli F, et al. Nonalcoholic fatty liver disease and risk of future cardiovascular events among type 2 diabetic patients. *Diabetes.* 2005;54(12):3541-3546.

11. Teli MR, James OF, Burt AD, et al. The natural history of nonalcoholic fatty liver: a follow-up study. *Hepatology.* 1995;22(6):1714-1719.

12. Fracanzani AL, Valenti L, Bugianesi E, et al. Risk of severe liver disease in nonalcoholic fatty liver disease with normal aminotransferase levels: a role for insulin resistance and diabetes. *Hepatology.* 2008;48(3):792-798.

13. Ratziu V, Giral P, Charlotte F, et al. Liver fibrosis in overweight patients. *Gastroenterology.* 2000;118(6):1117-1123.

14. Ratziu V, Massard J, Charlotte F, et al. Diagnostic value of biochemical markers (FibroTest-FibroSURE) for the prediction of liver fibrosis in patients with non-alcoholic fatty liver disease. *BMC Gastroenterol.* 2006;6:6.

15. Angulo P, Hui JM, Marchesini G, et al. The NAFLD fibrosis score: a noninvasive system that identi-fies liver fibrosis in patients with NAFLD. *Hepatology.* 2007;45(4):846-854.

16. Harrison SA, Oliver D, Arnold HL, et al. Development and validation of a simple NAFLD clinical scoring system for identifying patients without advanced disease. *Gut.* 2008;57(10):1441-1447.

17. Guha IN, Parkes J, Roderick P, et al. Noninvasive markers of fibrosis in nonalcoholic fatty liver disease: validating the European Liver Fibrosis Panel and exploring simple markers. *Hepatology.* 2008;47(2):455-460.

18. Cales P, Laine F, Boursier J, et al. Comparison of blood tests for liver fibrosis specific or not to NAFLD. *J Hepatol.* 2009;50(1):165-173.

19. Myers RP. Noninvasive diagnosis of nonalcoholic fatty liver disease. *Ann Hepatol.* 2009;8(Suppl):S25-S33.

20. Neuschwander-Tetri BA, Clark JM, Bass NM, et al. Clinical, laboratory and histological associations in adults with nonalcoholic fatty liver disease. *Hepatology.* 2010;52(3):913-924.

21. Saadeh S, Younossi ZM, Remer EM, et al. The utility of radiological imaging in nonalcoholic fatty liver disease. *Gastroenterology.* 2002;123(3):745-750.

22. Castera L. Non-invasive diagnosis of steatosis and fibrosis. *Diabetes Metab.* 2008;34(6):674-679.

23. Wong VW, Vergniol J, Wong GL. Diagnosis of fibrosis and cirrhosis using liver stiffness measure-ment in nonalcoholic fatty liver disease. *Hepatology.* 2010;51(2):454-462.

24. Foucher J, Castera L, Bernard PH, et al. Prevalence and factors associated with failure of liver stiff-ness measurement using FibroScan in a prospective study of 2114 examinations. *Eur J Gastroenterol Hepatol.* 2006;18(4):411-412.

25. Rafiq N, Bai C, Fang Y, et al. Long-term follow-up of patients with nonalcoholic fatty liver. *Clin Gastroenterol Hepatol.* 2009;7(2):234-238.

26. Sanyal AJ, Chalasani N, Kowdley KV, et al. Pioglitazone, vitamin E, or placebo for nonalcoholic steatohepatitis. *N Engl J Med.* 2010;362(18):1675-1685.

27. Mathurin P, Hollebecque A, Arnalsteen L, et al. Prospective study of the long-term effects of bariatric surgery on liver injury in patients without advanced disease. *Gastroenterology.* 2009;137(2):532-540.

28. Wong VW, Wong GL, Choi PC, et al. Disease progression of non-alcoholic fatty liver disease: a prospective study with paired liver biopsies at 3 years. *Gut.* 2010;59(7)969-974.

29. Seeff LB, Everson GT, Morgan TR, et al. Complication rate of percutaneous liver biopsies among persons with advanced chronic liver disease in the HALT-C trial. *Clin Gastroenterol Hepatol.* 2010;8(10):877-883.

30. Ratziu V, Charlotte F, Heurtier A, et al. Sampling variability of liver biopsy in nonalcoholic fatty liver disease. *Gastroenterology.* 2005;128(7):1898-1906.

31. Brunt EM. Pathology of fatty liver disease. *Mod Pathol.* 2007;20(Suppl):S40-S48.

32. Matteoni CA, Younossi ZM, Gramlich T, et al. Nonalcoholic fatty liver disease: a spectrum of clinical and pathological severity. *Gastroenterology.* 1999;116(6):1413-1419.

33. Brunt EM, Janney CG, Di Bisceglie AM, et al. Nonalcoholic steatohepatitis: a proposal for grading and staging the histological lesions. *Am J Gastroenterol.* 1999;94(9):2467-2474.

34. Kleiner DE, Brunt EM, Van Natta M, et al. Design and validation of a histological scoring system for nonalcoholic fatty liver disease. *Hepatology.* 2005;41(6):1313-1321.

35. Fukusato T, Fukushima J, Shiga J, et al. Interobserver variation in the histopathological assessment of nonalcoholic steatohepatitis. *Hepatol Res.* 2005;33(2):122-127.

36. Younossi ZM, Gramlich T, Liu YC, et al. Nonalcoholic fatty liver disease: assessment of variability in pathologic interpretations. *Mod Pathol.* 1998;11(6):560-565.

37. Vuppalanchi R, Unalp A, Van Natta ML, et al. Effects of liver biopsy sample length and number of readings on sampling variability in nonalcoholic fatty liver disease. *Clin Gastroenterol Hepatol.* 2009;7(4):481-486.

38. Bejarano PA, Koehler A, Sherman KE. Second opinion pathology in liver biopsy interpretation. *Am J Gastroenterol.* 2001;96(11):3158-3164.

39. Bravo AA, Sheth SG, Chopra S. Liver biopsy. *N Engl J Med.* 2001;344(7):495-500.

40. Goldstein NS, Hastah F, Galan MV, et al. Fibrosis heterogeneity in nonalcoholic steatohepatitis and hepatitis C virus needle core biopsy specimens. *Am J Clin Pathol.* 2005;123(3):382-387.

41. Merriman RB, Ferrell LD, Patti MG, et al. Correlation of paired liver biopsies in morbidly obese patients with suspected nonalcoholic fatty liver disease. *Hepatology.* 2006;44(4):874-880.

42. Piccinino F, Sagnelli E, Pasquale G, et al. Complications following percutaneous liver biopsy: A multicentre retrospective study on 68,276 biopsies. *J Hepatol.* 1986;2(2):165-173.

43. Janes CH, Lindor KD. Outcome of patients hospitalized for complications after outpatient liver biopsy. *Ann Intern Med.* 1993;118(2):96-98.

44. Perrault J, McGill DB, Ott BJ, et al. Liver biopsy: complications in 1000 inpatients and outpatients. *Gastroenterology.* 1978;74(1):103-106.

45. Eisenberg E, Konopniki M, Veitsman E, et al. Prevalence and characteristics of pain induced by percutaneous liver biopsy. *Anesth Analg.* 2003;96(5):1392-1396.

46. McAfee JH, Keeffe EB, Lee RG, et al. Transjugular liver biopsy. *Hepatology.* 1992;15(4):726-732.

47. Crockett SD, Kaltenbach T, Keeffe EB. Do we still need a liver biopsy? Are the serum fibrosis tests ready for prime time? *Clin Liver Dis.* 2006;10(3):513-534.

48. Halfon P, Munteanu M, Poynard T. FibroTest-ActiTest as a non-invasive marker of liver fibrosis. *Gastroenterol Clin Biol.* 2008;32(6Suppl):22-39.

49. Shah AG, Lydecker A, Murray K, et al. Comparison of noninvasive markers of fibrosis in patients with nonalcoholic fatty liver disease. *Clin Gastroenterol Hepatol.* 2009;7(10):1104-1112.

50. Yilmaz Y, Kedrah AE, Ozdogan O. Cytokeratin-18 fragments and biomarkers of the metabolic syndrome in nonalcoholic steatohepatitis. *World J Gastroenterol.* 2009;15(35):4387-4391.

51. Tsutsui M, Tanaka N, Kawakubo M, et al. Serum fragmented cytokeratin 18 levels reflect the histologic activity score of nonalcoholic fatty liver disease more accurately than serum alanine aminotransferase levels. *J Clin Gastroenterol.* 2010;44(6):440-447.

52. Wieckowska A, Zein NN, Yerian LM, et al. In vivo assessment of liver cell apoptosis as a novel biomarker of disease severity in nonalcoholic fatty liver disease. *Hepatology.* 2006;44(1):27-33.

53. Yilmaz Y, Dolar E, Ulukaya E, et al. Soluble forms of extracellular cytokeratin 18 may differentiate simple steatosis from nonalcoholic steatohepatitis. *World J Gastroenterol.* 2007;13(6):837-844.

54. Cassidy FH, Yokoo T, Aganovic L, et al. Fatty liver disease: MR imaging techniques for the detection and quantification of liver steatosis. *Radiographics.* 2009;29(1):231-260.

55. Ehman RL. Science to practice: can MR elastography be used to detect early steatohepatitis in fatty liver disease? *Radiology.* 2009;253(1):1-3.

56. Cho SG, Kim MY, Kim HJ, et al. Chronic hepatitis: in vivo proton MR spectroscopic evaluation of the liver and correlation with histopathologic findings. *Radiology.* 2001;221(3):740-746.

57. Clark JM. Weight loss as a treatment for nonalcoholic fatty liver disease. *J Clin Gastroenterol.* 2006;(40Suppl1):S39-S43.

58. Ueno T, Sugawara H, Sujaku K, et al. Therapeutic effects of restricted diet and exercise in obese patients with fatty liver. *J Hepatol.* 1997;27(1):103-107.

59. Miller ER 3rd, Pastor-Barriuso R, Dalal D, et al. Meta-analysis: high-dosage vitamin E supplementation may increase all-cause mortality. *Ann Intern Med.* 2005;142(1):37-46.

60. Rinella ME, McCarthy R, Thakrar K, et al. Dual-echo, chemical shift gradient-echo magnetic resonance imaging to quantify hepatic steatosis: implications for living liver donation. *Liver Transpl.* 2003;9(8):851-856.

61. Younossi ZM, Page S, Rafiq N, et al. A biomarker panel for non-alcoholic steatohepatitis (NASH) and NASH-related fibrosis. *Obes Surg.* 2011;21(4)431-439.

62. Ratziu V, Giral P, Munteanu M, et al. Screening for liver disease using non-invasive biomarkers (FibroTest, SteatoTest and NashTest) in patients with hyperlipidaemia. *Aliment Pharmacol Ther.* 2007;25(2):207-218.

63. Friedrich-Rust M, Hadji-Hosseini H, Kriener S, et al. Transient elastography with a new probe for obese patients for non-invasive staging of non-alcoholic steatohepatitis. *Eur Radiol.* 2010;20(10):2390-2396.

64. Cales P, Boursier J, Chaigneau J, et al. Diagnosis of different liver fibrosis characteristics by blood tests in non-alcoholic fatty liver disease. *Liver Int.* 2010;30(9):1346-1354.

65. Cales P, Boursier J, Oberti F, et al. FibroMeters: a family of blood tests for liver fibrosis. *Gastroenterol Clin Biol.* 2008;32(6Suppl1):40-51.

66. Mofrad P, Contos MJ, Haque M, et al. Clinical and histologic spectrum of nonalcoholic fatty liver disease associated with normal ALT values. *Hepatology.* 2003;37(6):1286-1292.

67. Feldstein AE, Canbay A, Angulo P, et al. Hepatocyte apoptosis and fas expression are prominent features of human nonalcoholic steatohepatitis. *Gastroenterology.* 2003;125(2):437-443.

68. Feldstein AE, Wieckowska A, Lopez AR, et al. Cytokeratin-18 fragment levels as noninvasive biomarkers for nonalcoholic steatohepatitis: a multicenter validation study. *Hepatology.* 2009;50(4):1072-1078.

69. Skelly MM, James PD, Ryder SD. Findings on liver biopsy to investigate abnormal liver function tests in the absence of diagnostic serology. *J Hepatol.* 2001;35(2):195-199.

CHAPTER 13

SHOULD THE HEPATIC VENOUS PRESSURE GRADIENT BE SEQUENTIALLY MEASURED TO MONITOR BETA-BLOCKER THERAPY IN THE PROPHYLAXIS OF VARICEAL HEMORRHAGE?

Cristina Ripoll, MD; Puneeta Tandon, MD; and Guadalupe Garcia-Tsao, MD

Variceal hemorrhage is a lethal complication of cirrhosis that results directly from portal hypertension. Therefore, reducing portal pressure through pharmacological therapy has been shown to result in a significant reduction in the probability of developing variceal hemorrhage. Since other complications of cirrhosis—such as ascites and encephalopathy—also result from portal hypertension, reduction in portal pressure also leads to a decreased development of these complications and a better survival rate. Nonselective beta-blockers (NSBB) are the key pharmacological therapy in the prevention of variceal hemorrhage. Because a significant reduction in portal pressure only occurs in about 40% of patients with cirrhosis on nonselective beta-blockers, it has been suggested that sequential portal pressure measurements (by assessment of the hepatic venous pressure gradient [HPVG]) to monitor the response to beta-blocker therapy should be performed to individualize therapy and improve outcomes. The advantages and disadvantages of such practice are discussed in this chapter.

Jensen D.
Controversies in Hepatology: The Experts Analyze Both Sides (pp 123-132)
© 2011 SLACK Incorporated

POINT

Assessing Patient Response to Pharmacological Therapy by Sequential Hepatic Venous Pressure Gradient Measurements Is the Rational Way to Treat Portal Hypertension

by Cristina Ripoll, MD

Nonselective beta-adrenergic blockers (NSBB) have been shown to prevent both the first variceal hemorrhage (primary prophylaxis) and recurrent variceal hemorrhage secondary prophylaxis in patients with cirrhosis.[1,2] Strong evidence has led to the recommendation of NSBB as first-line therapy for primary prophylaxis and of NSBB plus ligation as first-line therapy for secondary prophylaxis.[3,4]

NSBBs act by decreasing portal pressure both through a β-1 adrenergic blocking effect and, more importantly, through a β-2 blockade that allows unopposed alpha adrenergic splanchnic vasoconstriction. Accordingly, there is a lack of correlation between the reduction in heart rate, a β-1 effect, and the reduction in portal pressure. The recommendation is to adjust the dose of NSBB to the maximally tolerated dose or to a heart rate of 50 to 55 beats/minute, whichever occurs first. Rationally, however, the dose should be based on a portal pressure response rather than a heart rate response.

Nonselective Beta-Blockers Are Particularly Beneficial When Their Use Is Associated With a Reduction in Hepatic Venous Pressure Gradient

Hepatic venous pressure gradient (HVPG) is the best and most utilized method to estimate portal pressure. Studies of sequential HVPG measurements in patients on pharmacological therapy for either primary or secondary prophylaxis have provided important information. Patients in whom the HVPG is reduced to levels below 12 mm Hg are essentially protected from variceal hemorrhage,[5,6] while in those who demonstrate a reduction >20% from baseline the risk of recurrent hemorrhage is very low, in the order of 7% to 13%, which is the lowest rate of recurrent hemorrhage observed with any of the current therapies, including the transjugular intrahepatic portosystemic shunt.[6] Two meta-analyses summarize the 12 studies (4 primary prophylaxis, 8 secondary prophylaxis), that measured sequential HVPG during therapy to prevent variceal hemorrhage. They both show that patients who decrease HVPG to <12 mm Hg and/or >20% from baseline (ie, hemodynamic "responders") have not only a significantly lower rate of variceal hemorrhage but also a lower mortality.[7,8]

Studies suggest that in the setting of primary prophylaxis, a lower threshold HVPG reduction may be sufficient to prevent outcomes. In one of them, patients in whom HVPG decreased by >11% had a lower incidence of spontaneous bacterial peritonitis and bacteremia.[9] In a more recent study performed in patients with large varices who had never bled, those in whom HVPG decreased by >10% not only had a significantly lower rate of first variceal hemorrhage (5% versus 22% in 2 years), but also had a lower rate of ascites (23% versus 70%) and death (13% versus 27%).[10]

In secondary prophylaxis studies, traditional "responders" (ie, those in whom HVPG decreases to <12 mm Hg or >20% from baseline) are not only more likely to remain free of bleeding (72% versus 42% free of bleeding in nonresponders over 8 years of follow-up) but are also more likely to remain free of ascites (70% versus 42%), spontaneous bacterial peritonitis (94% versus 58%), hepatic encephalopathy (84% versus 58%), and death (survival probability 52% in nonresponders versus 95% in responders).[11]

Measuring Hepatic Venous Pressure Gradient Is Safe and Response Can Be Assessed in a Single Procedure

Many of the arguments against measuring HVPG are based on the notion that it is an invasive procedure with an inherent risk of complications that, additionally, would need to be performed twice in order to determine response to therapy.

The rate of complications associated with HVPG measurement reported in the literature is only in the order of 2.3% in 2364 patients,[12] with no fatalities reported in over 12,000 procedures.[13] Furthermore, most complications are associated to neck or groin hematomas, the development of which can be reduced with the use of ultrasound-guided venous puncture.[13]

Importantly, recent studies have demonstrated that measuring the acute response to an intravenous bolus of NSBB during a single HVPG procedure (0.15 mg/kg IV over 10 minutes with HVPG response assessed at minute 20) can also identify patients who will have a low bleeding rate in the long term.[10,14] This would forego the need to perform 2 HVPG measurements and would decrease potential morbidity and costs.

Knowledge of Hepatic Venous Pressure Gradient Response Can Improve Patient Management

NSBB has side effects that are significant enough to lead to treatment discontinuation in 15% of the cases and to limit the attainment of an appropriate dose. Knowledge of the hemodynamic response status—responder or nonresponder to NSBB—does not change the effect of a drug, but it may change physician and patient attitudes. In responders, it could improve patient adherence and could even lead to a greater tolerability of NSBB side effects. In nonresponders, it could lead to the addition of another pharmacological agent (eg, nitrates or carvedilol) that would improve the portal pressure-reducing effect of NSBB or to a change in therapy (eg, ligation).

Summary

Sequential HVPG measurements in patients with cirrhosis on NSBB for primary or secondary prophylaxis of variceal hemorrhage provide important prognostic information and can be invaluable in guiding their management. On one hand, knowing that the patient is a responder can further reinforce the motivation of the patient to continue on NSBB. On the other hand, the identification of nonresponders could lead to the administration of more effective therapies prior to the development of a clinical failure (eg, variceal hemorrhage).

KEY POINTS

- HVPG responders have many clinical benefits, including increased survival.
- Nonresponders can receive other therapeutic approaches early on.
- HVPG measurement is easily performed and has a low complication rate.
- Knowledge of HVPG response status can improve patient compliance and management.

COUNTERPOINT

There Is Not Enough Data to Support the Routine Use of Hepatic Venous Pressure Gradient for Monitoring Pharmacological Treatment of Portal Hypertension

by Puneeta Tandon, MD

There is no question that portal pressure reduction, determined by sequential HVPG measurements, is associated with a reduction in variceal hemorrhage, other complications of portal hypertension, and even death.[7] However, beyond its prognostic value, it is an invasive procedure, and unless the information gained through its practice can lead to a change in management, it would be difficult to recommend its use outside of clinical trials.

Hemodynamic Response Does Not Correlate Strongly Enough With Clinical Response

Although a large majority of hemodynamic responders are protected from variceal hemorrhage (only 10% will bleed), not all hemodynamic nonresponders will experience a variceal hemorrhage (up to 48% will bleed).[7,15] Accordingly, and as recently discussed, the percentage of patients free of hemorrhage is consistently higher than the rate of hemodynamic responders,[15] indicating a protective effect of pharmacological therapy that goes beyond hemodynamic response. In fact, in a study that measured variceal pressure (the factor that leads to variceal rupture), some patients that were considered HVPG nonresponders had an effective decrease in variceal pressure (and a similar reduction in variceal hemorrhage) presumably through a decrease in flow through the collateral system.[16] A study performed in rats with partial constriction of the portal vein showed that propranolol led to a reduction in portal blood flow of 32% that was

Table 13-1.					
STUDIES ON HEPATIC VENOUS PRESSURE GRADIENT-GUIDED THERAPY					
AUTHOR	INITIAL TREATMENT	N (TYPE OF PROPHYLAXIS)	BLEEDING IN RESPONDERS	RESCUE THERAPY IN NR	BLEEDING IN "RESCUED" NR
Bureau	BB ± ISMN	20 (primary)	0/14 (0%)	BB + ISMN	2/6 (33%)
	BB ± ISMN	14 (secondary)	2/6 (33%)	EVL	7/8 (88%)
Gonzalez	BB + ISMN	42 (secondary)	3/24 (12%)	EVL drug* TIPS**	2/10 (20%) 0/8 (0%)
Villanueva[†]	BB + ISMN or Prazosin	27 (secondary)	3/20 (15%)	None	4/7 (57%)

NR = nonresponders; BB = beta-blockers; ISMN = isosorbide mononitrate; EVL = endoscopic variceal ligation; TIPS = transjugular intrahepatic portosystemic shunt

* in partial responders; ** in total nonresponders, † randomized controlled trial

accompanied by a reduction in portal pressure of only 18%, which is disproportionately small because of a concomitant rise in portal-collateral vascular resistance accompanying the portal blood flow reduction.[17] A reduction in collateral flow would include a decreased blood flow and thereby a decreased pressure through gastroesophageal collaterals (ie, varices), a beneficial effect.

Hepatic Venous Pressure Gradient-Guided Therapy Has Not Been Shown to Improve Outcomes

Even when assessment of an HVPG response can identify patients at a higher risk of failing first-line pharmacological therapy, a therapeutic strategy that would improve outcomes in nonresponders has not yet been established. As shown in Table 13-1, studies using HVPG-guided therapy have included only a small number of patients and only one of them is a randomized controlled trial. In the first study by Bureau et al[18] that included patients treated for both primary and secondary prophylaxis, rescue therapies did not improve outcomes. In fact, in the secondary prophylaxis group a switch to endoscopic variceal ligation (EVL) resulted in a very high rebleeding rate. The study by González et al describes a strategy that resulted in very low rebleeding rates (11%)[19] in nonresponders. Partial nonresponders (HVPG reduction between 10% to 20%) received EVL in addition to NSBB, while total nonresponders (HVPG reduction <10%) received transjugular intrahepatic portosystemic shunt (TIPS) therapy. Unfortunately, the study did not include a control group managed in a standard fashion. In the only randomized controlled trial,[20] Villanueva et al compared HVPG-guided therapy to standard therapy with EVL plus nadolol in the prevention of recurrent variceal hemorrhage. Even though they demonstrate that responders have a significantly lower rebleeding rate than nonresponders (74% versus 32%, $P<0.01$), ultimately the rebleeding rate in patients randomized to HVPG-guided therapy (22%) was not significantly different from that in the EVL plus nadolol group (23%). This may have been due to the fact that no rescue therapy was provided to nonresponders.

Hepatic Venous Pressure Gradient Is an Invasive Procedure With Potential Side Effects and Cost Effectiveness Data Are Limited

Although HVPG is a relatively safe procedure, it is still an invasive procedure and has inherent risks even if only one measurement is performed. It requires conscious sedation, exposure to an intravenous radiological contrast agent, placement of a central venous line, and passage of a guide wire and catheter through the right atrium. Major complications have occurred, including supraventricular arrhythmias and local injury at the venous puncture site (leakage, hematoma, and rarely arteriovenous fistulae or Horner syndrome). Additionally, the cost of the procedure may be considered another setback, and in the absence of proven effectiveness of HVPG-guided therapy and the optimal rescue therapy for nonresponders, cost-effectiveness analyses are irrelevant.

KEY POINTS

- Beta-blocker therapy may have beneficial effects in preventing variceal hemorrhage that goes beyond the hemodynamic portal pressure-reducing effect.
- Evidence is lacking regarding a higher efficacy of HVPG-guided therapy compared to standard therapy.

EXPERT OPINION

Measuring Portal Pressure Is a Rational Method to Assess Response to Pharmacological Therapy of Portal Hypertension

by Guadalupe Garcia-Tsao, MD

In the same way that measuring arterial pressure is key in the management of arterial hypertension, measuring portal pressure by the HVPG should be key in the pharmacological management of portal hypertension. Determining the response rate (ie, the degree of reduction in HVPG after pharmacological therapy) has been shown to be useful not only in identifying patients at a low risk of developing variceal hemorrhage, but also in identifying patients at a lower risk of developing other complications of cirrhosis, including death.[10,11] HVPG reduction can occur spontaneously or, more frequently, after treatment with NSBB with or without the addition of nitrates. The "responder" rate is 37% with NSBB alone and 44% when nitrates are associated.[20] Obviously, if a therapy was available that would yield a responder rate in the order of 90% to 100%, HVPG monitoring would not be necessary; however, this is unlikely to occur anytime soon. While measuring HVPG is an absolute requirement in any clinical trial on portal hypertension involving pharmacological therapy,[12] there are various issues outlined below that require resolution before HVPG-guided therapy can be widely recommended in daily practice.

Timing/Need for a Second Hepatic Venous Pressure Gradient Measurement

Most studies on HVPG response have been performed in the setting of secondary prophylaxis (ie, patients that have recovered from an episode of variceal hemorrhage) with repeat HVPG performed 30 to 120 days after initiation of pharmacological therapy. They demonstrate that patients in whom the HVPG is reduced below a certain threshold have a very low risk of developing recurrent variceal hemorrhage. With longer time intervals between HVPG measurements, the predictive value of HVPG reduction is much lower[7] and therefore the second measurement should take place as soon as the maximum tolerated dose of the drug(s) is reached. Recent retrospective studies have demonstrated that the acute HVPG response assessed 20 minutes after the administration of intravenous propranolol is a good predictor of first variceal hemorrhage[10] and recurrent variceal hemorrhage.[14] Although this may be a more cost-effective strategy than the evaluation of a chronic HVPG response, it requires further validation, particularly in the setting of primary prophylaxis where acute HVPG response has not uniformly shown to significantly predict first variceal hemorrhage.[14]

Threshold of Hepatic Venous Pressure Gradient Reduction That Defines a Good Response

The threshold decrease in HVPG that defines hemodynamic response is a decrease in HVPG to values below 12 mm Hg or a decrease >20% from baseline.[7,8] Notably, in studies performed in compensated cirrhosis, a lower chronic response threshold (a decrease >10% from baseline) has been shown to reduce the development of varices (pre-primary prophylaxis),[21] first variceal hemorrhage,[10] ascites, and death.[10] In acute response studies, the threshold appears to also be lower at 10%[10] or 12%.[14] These lower thresholds in the definition of response require further validation.

Treatment in Hemodynamic Nonresponders

The best management strategy for nonresponders remains to be determined in the setting of clinical trials. Nonresponders to pharmacological therapy appear not to benefit from additional endoscopic therapy.[18,22] So far, studies of HVPG-guided therapy are uncontrolled or show no differences compared to standard therapy.[18,19,23] It will be important to identify predictors of bleeding among hemodynamic nonresponders because this will allow for further risk stratification and the application (or not) of rational rescue therapies. As recently shown, clinical parameters such as Child-Pugh class and red wale marks on varices appear to be better predictors of first variceal hemorrhage than the acute hemodynamic response.[14]

Standardization of the Hepatic Venous Pressure Gradient Measurement Method

It is essential that HVPG measurements be performed according to recently described standards.[13,24] Measurements done without using the appropriate technique can lead to more confusion than helpful information. At the recent Baveno consensus conference, it was recommended that "in centers where adequate resources and expertise are available, HVPG measurements should be routinely used for prognostic and therapeutic indications."[25] In centers where the procedure is not routinely utilized and where it is performed by interventional radiologists without the intervention of trained hepatologists, as occurs in most centers in the United States, there is an increased chance of obtaining suboptimal results by a faulty technique (eg, not using a balloon catheter or using monitor readings rather than paper or electronic tracings).[12] In such centers, standardization of the technique, formal certification, and quality assessment are needed before the HVPG can be utilized as a routine clinical tool.

Summary

While NSBB continues to be first-line therapy in the prophylaxis of variceal hemorrhage and while NSBBs are particularly beneficial in patients in whom portal pressure is reduced, many questions remain to be resolved before the sequential measurement of HVPG to assess response to beta-blocker therapy can be widely recommended for clinical use.

References

1. D'Amico G, Pagliaro L, Bosch J. Pharmacological treatment of portal hypertension: an evidence-based approach. *Sem Liv Dis*. 1999;19:475-505.
2. Bernard B, Lebrec D, Mathurin P, et al. Beta-adrenergic antagonists in the prevention of gastrointestinal rebleeding in patients with cirrhosis: a meta-analysis. *Hepatology*. 1997;25:63-70.
3. Garcia-Tsao G, Sanyal AJ, Grace ND, et al. Prevention and management of gastroesophageal varices and variceal hemorrhage in cirrhosis. *Hepatology*. 2007;46:922-938.
4. Garcia-Tsao G, Bosch J. Management of varices and variceal hemorrhage in cirrhosis. *N Engl J Med*. 2010;362:823-832.
5. Groszmann RJ, Bosch J, Grace N, et al. Hemodynamic events in a prospective randomized trial of propranolol vs placebo in the prevention of the first variceal hemorrhage. *Gastroenterology*. 1990;99(5):1401-1407.
6. Bosch J, Garcia-Pagan JC. Prevention of variceal rebleeding. *Lancet*. 2003;361:952-954.
7. D'Amico G, Garcia-Pagan JC, Luca A, et al. HVPG reduction and prevention of variceal bleeding in cirrhosis. A systematic review. *Gastroenterology*. 2006;131:1611-1624.
8. Albillos A, Banares R, Gonzalez M, et al. Value of the hepatic venous pressure gradient to monitor drug therapy for portal hypertension: a meta-analysis. *Am J Gastroenterol*. 2007;102:1116-1126.
9. Turnes J, Garcia-Pagan JC, Abraldes JG, et al. Pharmacological reduction of portal pressure and long-term risk of first variceal bleeding in patients with cirrhosis. *Am J Gastroenterol*. 2006;101:506-512.
10. Villanueva C, Aracil C, Colomo A, et al. Acute hemodynamic response to beta-blockers and prediction of long-term outcome in primary prophylaxis of variceal bleeding. *Gastroenterology*. 2009,137:119-128.
11. Abraldes JG, Tarantino I, Turnes J, et al. Hemodynamic response to pharmacological treatment of portal hypertension and long-term prognosis of cirrhosis. *Hepatology*. 2003;37:902-908.
12. Garcia-Tsao G, Bosch J, Groszmann RJ. Portal hypertension and variceal bleeding--unresolved issues. Summary of an American Association for the Study of Liver Diseases and European Association for the Study of the Liver Single-Topic Conference. *Hepatology*. 2008;47:1764-1772.
13. Bosch J, Abraldes JG, Berzigotti A, et al. The clinical use of HVPG measurements in chronic liver disease. *Nat Rev Gastroenterol Hepatol*. 2009;6:573-582.
14. La Mura V, Abraldes JG, Raffa S, et al. Prognostic value of acute hemodynamic response to i.v. propranolol in patients with cirrhosis and portal hypertension. *J Hepatol*. 2009;51:279-287.
15. Thalheimer U, Bosch J, Burroughs AK. How to prevent varices from bleeding: shades of grey: the case for nonselective beta blockers. *Gastroenterology*. 2007;133:2029-2036.
16. Escorsell A, Bordas JM, Castaneda B, et al. Predictive value of the variceal pressure response to continued pharmacological therapy in patients with cirrhosis and portal hypertension. *Hepatology*. 2000;31:1061-1067.

17. Kroeger RJ Groszmann RJ. Increased portal venous resistance hinders portal pressure reduction during the administration of beta-adrenergic blocking agents in a portal hypertensive model. *Hepatology.* 1985;5:97-101.
18. Bureau C, Peron JM, Alric L, et al. "A la carte" treatment of portal hypertension: adapting medical therapy to hemodynamic response for the prevention of bleeding. *Hepatology.* 2002;36:1361-1366.
19. Gonzalez A, Augustin S, Perez M, et al. Hemodynamic response-guided therapy for prevention of variceal rebleeding: an uncontrolled pilot study. *Hepatology.* 2006;44:806-812.
20. Miñano C, Garcia-Tsao G. Clinical pharmacology of portal hypertension. *Gastroenterol Clin North Am.* 2010;39(3):681-695.
21. Groszmann RJ, Garcia-Tsao G, Bosch J, et al. Beta-blockers to prevent gastroesophageal varices in patients with cirrhosis. *N Engl J Med.* 2005;353:2254-2261.
22. Garcia-Pagan JC, Villanueva C, Albillos A, et al. Nadolol plus isosorbide mononitrate alone or associated with band ligation in the prevention of variceal rebleeding: a multicenter randomized controlled trial. *Gut.* 2009;58:1144-1150.
23. Villanueva C, Aracil C, Colomo A, et al. Clinical trial: a randomized controlled study on prevention of variceal rebleeding comparing nadolol + ligation vs. hepatic venous pressure gradient-guided pharmacological therapy. *Aliment Pharmacol Ther.* 2009;29:397-408.
24. Groszmann RJ, Wongcharatrawee S. The hepatic venous pressure gradient: anything worth doing should be done right. *Hepatology.* 2004;39:280-283.
25. de Franchis R. Revising consensus in portal hypertension: report of the Baveno V consensus workshop on methodology of diagnosis and therapy in portal hypertension. *J Hepatol.* 2010;53:762-768.

CHAPTER 14

STANDARD DOSE OR AVOID URSODIOL THERAPY IN PRIMARY SCLEROSING CHOLANGITIS?

Dr. JS Halliday, MBBS (Hons.), FRACP; Ashley Barnabas, MD; and Roger W. Chapman, MD, FRCP

Primary sclerosing cholangitis (PSC) is a chronic progressive disorder which is characterized by inflammation, fibrosis, and stricturing of intrahepatic and extrahepatic bile ducts, ultimately leading to liver cirrhosis. The etiology is poorly understood; an immune-mediated basis is suggested by lymphocytic portal tract infiltration and close association with autoantibodies, human leukocyte antigen (HLA) haplotypes (HLA, B8, DR3, and DQ2), other autoimmune diseases, and inflammatory bowel disease.[1] It is not a classical autoimmune disease, however, with male predominance at a ratio of 2 to 1, and a poor response to immunosuppressive agents.

The main goals of therapy in PSC are retardation and reversal of the disease process and management of this progressive disease and its complications. Although the course is variable and unpredictable, PSC is generally progressive and leads to biliary cirrhosis. Liver failure, hepatobiliary, and colonic cancer are the major conditions that affect survival, malignancy becoming the most important cause of death over the last decade.

While the bile acid ursodeoxycholic acid (UDCA) is established for the medical treatment of primary biliary cirrhosis, its usefulness in PSC is less clear. The aim of this chapter is to examine the "pros and cons" of UDCA treatment in PSC.

Jensen D.
*Controversies in Hepatology: The Experts Analyze Both
Sides (pp 133-144)*
© 2011 SLACK Incorporated

Ursodeoxycholic Acid Is Indicated for the Treatment of Primary Sclerosing Cholangitis

by Dr. JS Halliday, MBBS (Hons.), FRACP

For more than 20 years, UDCA has been used extensively for the treatment of cholestatic liver conditions and is now the standard therapy for conditions such as primary biliary cirrhosis.[2]

In contrast, the use of UDCA remains controversial for PSC, a similarly chronic and progressive cholestatic disease. PSC is characterized by inflammatory fibrosis and destruction of the biliary tree, leading to multifocal bile duct strictures and eventually cirrhosis in the majority of cases.[1]

Despite the controversy, there is clear evidence—both at a cellular level and in a broad range of clinical trials—that UDCA therapy is beneficial for PSC. Ultimately, its use continues to be questioned for two reasons. First, there is a lack of definitive evidence that UDCA improves survival in PSC. Second, a recent trial comparing high-dose UDCA to placebo resulted in increased adverse outcomes in the treatment arm.[3] At face value, these reasons are misleading because they serve only to highlight the difficulty in interpreting evidence for rare conditions like PSC that evolve slowly and for which accurate markers of disease progression are lacking.

Mechanism of Action

UDCA is a hydrophilic, secondary bile acid that is naturally produced in mammals when intestinal bacteria metabolize primary bile acids.

At a pathophysiological level, UDCA is an appealing treatment choice for PSC because it targets a number of the mechanisms by which cellular injury occurs in cholestatic liver disease. As a cholerectic agent, UDCA reduces exposure to hepatotoxic bile salts by increasing outflow of bile from the liver.[4] Studies from the early 1990s demonstrated that UDCA also has a direct cytoprotective effect on hepatocytes and inhibits apoptosis.[5] UDCA also exerts a cytoprotective effect indirectly by displacing hydrophobic, hepatotoxic bile acids from the bile acid pool.[6] Finally, UDCA has been shown to act as an immunomodulator by suppressing cytokine and immunoglobulin production. Given that, at least in part, PSC results from immune dysregulation, this effect may be important in altering disease progression.

Protection Against Disease Progression

A number of controlled and uncontrolled studies have consistently demonstrated that, at a wide range of doses, UDCA improves liver biochemistry (Table 14-1).

Demonstrating that biochemical changes translate into an improvement in disease progression in large controlled trials has been difficult, although several small pilot studies using surrogate markers suggested efficacy of UDCA. Lindor et al published the earliest substantial trial in 1997.[7] This double-blind, placebo-controlled trial recruited 105 patients and treated them with a dose of 13 to 15 mg/kg/day of UDCA for 2 years. An improvement in serum liver tests was demonstrated but there was no clear improvement in symptoms or liver histology observed.

Table 14-1.

SELECTED TRIALS OF URSODEOXYCHOLIC ACID FOR TREATMENT OF PRIMARY SCLEROSING CHOLANGITIS

AUTHOR	YEAR	PTS	DOSE UDCA/ DAY	TRIAL TYPE	TRIAL PERIOD (MONTHS)	LIVER FUNCTION TESTS	SYMPTOMS IMPROVED	LIVER HISTOLOGY IMPROVED
Beuers[5]	1992	6	13 to 15 mg/kg	Double-blind, placebo controlled	12	Improved	N	Y
Stichl[10]	1994	20	750 mg	Double-blind, placebo controlled	12 to 48	Improved	N	Y
Lindor[7]	1997	105	13 to 15 mg/kg	Double-blind, placebo controlled	34	Improved	N	N
Mitchell[11]	2001	26	20 to 25 mg/kg	Double-blind, placebo controlled	24	Improved	N	Y
Harnois[12]	2001	30	25 to 30 mg/kg	Open label	12	Improved	Not done	Not done
Okolicsanyi[13]	2003	86	8 to 13 mg/kg	Open label, placebo controlled	120	Improved	Y	N
Olsson[8]	2005	110	17 to 23 mg/kg	Double-blind, placebo controlled	60	Improved	N	Not done
Lindor[3]	2009	150	25 to 30 mg/kg	Double-blind, placebo controlled	60	Improved	N	N

The second large, double-blind, placebo-controlled UDCA study from Scandanavia enrolled 219 patients using a higher UDCA dose of 17 to 23 mg/kg/day for 5 years.[8] A strong trend toward increased survival in the UDCA group compared with placebo was observed but, unfortunately, due to significantly fewer endpoints than expected (death or liver transplantation), the study was insufficiently powered to produce a statistically significant result. Questions have also been raised about adequate patient compliance in this trial because, unlike earlier studies, biochemical responses in the UDCA treatment arm were unexpectedly poor.

Table 14-2.
DIFFICULTIES STUDYING PRIMARY SCLEROSING CHOLANGITIS
■ Rare, insidiously progressive disease; difficult to recruit patients and long follow-up time required.
■ Absence of reliable markers for assessing disease progression.
■ Highly variable disease course.
■ Comorbid pathology—Cholangiocarcinoma, choledocolithiasis, biliary sludge influence prognosis, and progression.

The difficulty obtaining a statistically significant improvement in survival in these trials is not surprising given the fact that the typical median transplantation-free survival for patients with PSC is 18 years.[9] The insidious progression of PSC is not the only factor, however, that makes it difficult to design and carry out trials to demonstrate a survival benefit with UDCA therapy (Table 14-2). The rarity of PSC makes recruitment difficult and, like the Scandinavian trial, most studies have been subsequently underpowered.

Unfortunately, the lack of reliable, noninvasive markers for disease progression also adds to the difficulty of studying this disease. Prognostic models such as the Mayo PSC Risk Score have been shown to correlate with survival but have proven to be ineffective in predicting prognosis for the individual patient. Liver function tests may fluctuate significantly, independent of disease progression, due to coexisting pathology such as choledocholithiasis and biliary sludge. Additionally, the development of main duct strictures (up to 45% of patients) and cholangiocarcinoma (6% to 20% of patients) makes the disease course highly variable from patient to patient. Even when liver biopsies are used to assess disease progression, sampling variability can still produce unreliable results.

Chemoprotection Against Carcinogenesis

PSC is associated with an increased risk of cholangiocarcinoma, gallbladder cancer, colorectal cancer, and possibly pancreatic cancer.[14] At least for colonic dysplasia and cancer, both at a cellular and clinical level, UDCA has been shown to reduce this risk. At present, this is perhaps the most persuasive reason for using UDCA to treat PSC.

The mechanism by which UDCA acts to reduce cancer risk is poorly understood but, at least in vitro, UDCA has been demonstrated to inhibit growth stimulated by deoxycholic acid in a number of tumor cell lines.[15]

Three quarters of PSC patients of Northern European descent have coexisting inflammatory bowel disease (IBD), usually total ulcerative colitis. This group (PSC/IBD) is at an even higher risk of colorectal cancer than those who have IBD alone.[16] Some studies have suggested the risk for colonic dysplasia or cancer in patients with PSC/IBD approaches 50% after 25 years of colitis.[17]

UDCA has been demonstrated in 3 clinical studies to reduce rates of colonic dysplasia and colorectal cancer. A cross-sectional study examined 59 patients with PSC/ ulcerative colitis (UC) enrolled in their colonoscopic surveillance program.[17] and demonstrated a significant reduction in rates of high-grade dysplasia (and rates of dysplasia) in patients taking UDCA compared with those who were not. (High grade: odds ratio 0.16 [95% CI, 0.03 to 0.96], $P = 0.04$). Pardi et al[17,18] followed 52 patients for 355 patient years in a randomized, placebo-controlled trial and also found a significant reduction in dysplasia and cancer numbers in the UDCA group. A third historical cohort study showed a nonsignificant reduction in the incidence of colorectal dysplasia and cancer in patients taking UDCA compared with those who were not, but no data on the use of other potentially protective drugs such as 5-aminosalysilic acids were collected.[19]

Cholangiocarcinoma occurs in 6% to 20% of patients with PSC. Unfortunately, up to 50% of these cholangiocarcinomas are discovered within the first year of the diagnosis of PSC.[20] The likely explanation for this is that it is actually the development of symptomatic cholangiocarcinoma that brings some patients with previously unrecognized PSC to medical attention. In light of this, the beneficial effect of UDCA in preventing cholangiocarcinoma is understandably more difficult to prove. Nevertheless, a retrospective study by Brandsaeter et al[21] that examined hepatobiliary cancers in a PSC population referred for transplantation found reduced rates of cancer in patients receiving UDCA.

High-Dose Ursodeoxycholic Acid

Until recently, no significant adverse effects had been reported with the use of UDCA. Two small pilot studies looking at high-dose UDCA showed that high doses are well tolerated and effective.[12,22] A recent trial by Lindor and colleagues has, however, brought this into question.[3] This double-blind, controlled study was terminated prematurely because of an increased risk of serious adverse events (development of cirrhosis, varices, death, or liver transplantation) in patients treated with high-dose UDCA (28 to 30 mg/kg/day) compared with placebo.

A number of explanations have been proposed to explain this surprising result. It is possible that the benefit of UDCA may have been reduced because a large number of patients recruited already had advanced liver disease at enrollment.

Another possible explanation for the poor outcome in the recent trial is that high doses of UDCA may allow unabsorbed drug to enter the colon and subsequently be modified into hepatotoxic bile acids, such as lithocholic acid. A previous study by Rost et al[23] demonstrated that biliary enrichment of UDCA plateaus at 22 to 25 mg/kg. Indeed, the hypothesis that excess UDCA may result in production of hepatotoxic bile acids is supported by recent data examining baseline and end of treatment serum bile acid levels in patients from the high-dose trial. Markedly elevated serum lithocholic acid levels were found in patients treated with UDCA compared with those who received only placebo.[24]

Other possibilities are that decreased apoptosis of hepatic stellate cells may have led to increased fibrogenesis, and lastly, the relatively small number of primary outcomes reached may have led to a chance finding.

Summary

At a dose of 15 to 23 mg/kg/day, UDCA has been proven to be safe and beneficial in the treatment of PSC. There are convincing data that it improves liver biochemistry and may reduce the risk of dysplasia and cancer in the colon in patients with PSC/IBD. Data demonstrating an absolute benefit on transplant-free survival are inconclusive. Rather than indicating an absence of therapeutic benefit, however, this results from the difficulty of obtaining such evidence in this rare and insidiously progressive disease.

KEY POINTS

- UDCA is a naturally occurring hydrophilic bile acid that displaces toxic hydrophobic bile acids from the bile acid pool.

- UDCA is of proven efficacy in the treatment of chronic cholestatic liver disorders such as PBC.

- Trials of moderate doses of UDCA (17 to 20 mg/kg/day) have shown a strong trend toward increased survival.

- UDCA probably exerts a chemoprotective effect against the increased risk of dysplasia/colorectal cancer that occurs in PSC patients with IBD.

COUNTERPOINT

Ursodeoxycholic Acid Should Not Be Used in the Treatment of Primary Sclerosing Cholangitis

by Ashley Barnabas, MD

Clinicians, understandably, are uncomfortable with not having any effective treatment for a disease that can be relentless in its course. In view of its efficacy in selected patients with primary biliary cirrhosis (PBC) and other cholestatic disorders, UDCA is intuitively an attractive potential therapeutic agent in the setting of PSC. It is well tolerated even in high doses[22] and improves biochemical parameters in most randomized controlled trials (RCTs) to date. It also has a number of theoretical benefits, both on PSC and neoplasia associated with PSC.

The evidence, however, is that UDCA is ineffective at standard to high doses (15 to 23 mg/kg) and potentially harmful at very high dosage (30 mg/kg). Although UDCA is commonly prescribed in the setting of PSC, the facts suggest that we are treating numbers by substituting improvements in biochemistry for objective measures of outcome. This therapeutic failure is well demonstrated in the epidemiological data, which show no improvement in the survival of patients over the past few decades. UDCA is an effective treatment in PBC[25] but has not been shown to be beneficial in PSC.

What Is the Evidence of Efficacy?

Chazouillères initially showed improvements in transaminases alkaline phosphatase (ALP) and gamma-glutamyl transferase (GGT) in 15 patients who received UDCA over a 6-month period, but no improvement in symptoms in this time.[26] A small, open label pilot study of 12 patients treated with 10 mg/kg over a 30-month interrupted period was then performed by O'Brien.[27] This demonstrated improvements in liver biochemistry and symptom scores. Both symptoms and biochemical parameters deteriorated in the off treatment phases of this trial. No attempt was made to establish long-term outcomes in these pilot studies and the placebo effect on symptoms, of course, could not be assessed.

The first prospective, double-blind, randomized trial of UDCA was performed by Beuers et al in 1991 in a group of 14 patients, with 6 in the treatment arm.[5] One patient withdrew from the study owing to UDCA-induced diarrhea. In the 5 remaining patients at 12 months, ALP, aspartate aminotransferase (AST), alanine transaminase (ALT), and bilirubin had improved. However, no change in hydrophobic bile acid concentrations was demonstrated. Liver histology was looked at as a marker of long-term outcome. A multi parametric scoring system, introduced previously in the setting of PBC[28]—rather than Ludwig's scoring system—was used in their analysis. Thus, although there was a significant difference in multi parametric scores, this was in a small group of patients with a scoring system not validated elsewhere. Paired liver biopsies were not used in this trial but later evidence suggests that this is a useful method of compensating for the wide sampling variability of PSC.[29]

In a much larger RCT,[7] 105 patients were recruited over a mean follow-up period of 2.2 years in a randomized, double-blind trial of UDCA at 13 to 15 mg/kg doses. Importantly, this trial set clinical outcomes as the primary end points. Again, improvements in serum ALP, AST, bilirubin, and albumin levels at 1 and 2 years were demonstrated, but neither adverse clinical outcomes nor liver histological findings were significantly affected by treatment with UDCA.

Has the Dose of Ursodiol Been Too Low?

After trials failed to show any change in outcome with UDCA, it was hypothesized that response to UDCA was a dose-dependent phenomenon. That UDCA is well tolerated even in a higher dose may at least partly explain the enthusiasm for the studies that followed. In 2001, Mitchell performed a randomized, placebo-controlled trial of UDCA 20 mg/kg in a total of 26 patients over a 2-year period.[11] In the small group of 13 patients treated with UDCA, absence of progression of disease on biopsy staging was significantly associated with UDCA treatment, but confidence intervals were wide and the authors acknowledged the limited value of this statistic in a small pilot trial of a heterogeneous group.

In 2005, Olsson published a RCT of 219 patients in which 110 were treated with 17 to 23 mg/kg of UDCA.[8] UDCA did not have any significant effect on the primary endpoint of death or transplantation. The incidence of cholangiocarcinoma was not significantly affected. There was no effect on pruritus and no significant change in self-report quality-of-life scores in the patients on UDCA. Interestingly, UDCA had no significant effect on ALP and no better outcome in patients whose liver biochemistry improved on UDCA (so-called UDCA responders). The authors commented that their study was underpowered to show a significant effect on the primary endpoint and there was a nonsignificant trend toward benefit in the UDCA group. This is primarily because 8 patients were transplanted in the non-UDCA group against 5 in the UDCA group. They do not, however, tell us how many patients met minimal listing criteria during the study period. This may be more useful, as it would be less likely to reflect confounding factors such as medical contraindications to transplantation or graft availability for blood groups.

The Effect of Higher Doses of Ursodeoxycholic Acid?

These disappointing results led various authors to conclude that it was not that UDCA was ineffective, but rather that it was not being used in a sufficient dose.

Cullen et al examined the use of UDCA in 31 patients with PSC.[22] All were treated for 2 years at a dose of 10, 20, or 30 mg. Liver biopsies were obtained in 23 patients and were included in the per protocol analysis. One of 9 patients in the 10 mg/kg group had a significant improvement in Ludwig score of 2. One of 6 patients in the 30 mg/kg group had a Ludwig score that deteriorated significantly by 3. Overall there was no demonstrable effect of high-dose UDCA on histology. Mayo PSC Risk Scores were also calculated in both patient groups. This multi-parametric scoring system incorporates age, serum bilirubin, AST, albumin, and a history of variceal bleeding. The 20 mg/kg and 30 mg/kg dose UDCA groups tended to have a greater reduction in Mayo PSC Risk Score, but the investigators did not comment on the extent to which this improvement could be attributed to UDCA's already well established effects on liver biochemistry. The improvement in Mayo PSC Risk Score only achieved statistical significance in the 30 mg/kg group. This was surprising, as Rost had previously been thought to have demonstrated that UDCA concentration in bile plateaus at a dose of 22 to 25 mg/kg.[23]

Shi identified 8 RCTs with a total of 465 patients examining UDCA (dose range 10 to 23 mg/kg) in PSC in a meta-analysis in 2008.[30] The analysis concluded that there was no benefit on survival-free rate of transplantation. Furthermore, no effect on symptom control was shown. All trials showed improvements in liver biochemistry, but this did not appear to translate into any clinical benefit.

Even Higher Dose of Ursodeoxycholic Acid?

Shi's meta-analysis predated the most recent RCT of very high-dose UDCA (28 to 30 mg/kg).[6] An initial pilot study of 30 patients had suggested that very high-dose UDCA was generally well tolerated and led to an improvement in the Mayo PSC Risk Score.[12] In light of this, 150 patients were randomized to receive either a very high dose (28 to 30 mg/kg) UDCA or placebo for 5 years. The primary outcomes measured were cirrhosis, varices, cholangiocarcinoma, liver transplantation, or death. The study was terminated at 6 years because it found that, compared with placebo, very high-dose UDCA was associated with a 2.3 times increased risk of a primary endpoint, after adjustment for baseline risk stratification. Once again, improvements in liver biochemistry did not result in an improved outcome. As this study was terminated prematurely, only 31 of the 150 patients enrolled had liver biopsies on completion of 5 years of treatment; no significant differences in Ludwig score could be demonstrated.

Small Duct Primary Sclerosing Cholangitis

Charatcharoenwitthaya et al performed a longitudinal cohort study on 42 patients with small duct PSC over a 62-month mean follow-up period.[31] Thirty of these were treated with UDCA for at least 1 year, 7 did not receive UDCA, and 5 were excluded from the analysis as they underwent transplantation within 1 year of enrolling in the study. In concordance with the previous work, improvements in AST and ALP were seen over a 2-year period, but UDCA was not shown to have a significant effect on disease progression. Thus, there is no evidence to suggest that UDCA is of benefit in the treatment of small duct PSC.

Ursodeoxycholic Acid and Chemoprevention

It has been suggested that UDCA may help to prevent the development of colorectal neoplasia. This is potentially of great importance given the increased risk of dysplasia and colorectal cancer in PSC-associated colitis.

In reality, the available data are generally retrospective and comparisons with other potentially chemoprotective agents such as mesalazine are not made. In a retrospective study of 59 patients with PSC undergoing surveillance colonoscopy at the University of Washington, Tung concluded that UDCA was associated with a low prevalence of colonic dysplasia.[17] Forty-one of the group studied were on UDCA prior to entry into the study. The groups were heterogeneous, with those not on UDCA significantly more likely to be male and to have a younger onset of colitis. They concluded that the group on UDCA was less likely to develop colonic dysplasia. However, the result failed to achieve significance when biopsies indefinite for dysplasia were excluded from the analysis and multivariate adjustments were made for the heterogeneity of the patient groups. The reasons for patients being selected for UDCA treatment was not made clear. An earlier historical cohort study in 132 patients with PSC did not identify UDCA use as being protective against colonic dysplasia.[32]

Pardi conversely suggested in a retrospective analysis that UDCA does indeed protect against colonic dysplasia.[8,18] This may indeed be the case, but it is simply an assumption that UDCA has any superiority over nonsteroidal anti-inflammatory drugs (NSAIDs) or 5-ASA compounds as a chemoprotective agent. Further prospective data are required to clarify whether this potential effect is genuine.

Thirty-three percent to 50% of cholangiocarcinomas follow within 1 year of the diagnosis of PSC. This implies that many cholangiocarcinomas predate the clinical diagnosis of PSC. Any chemopreventive strategy, therefore, may be limited in efficacy. Indeed, UDCA in Olsson's study did not affect the development of cholangiocarcinoma.[8]

Is There Epidemiological Evidence of Efficacy?

Epidemiological data reflect the lack of any effective drug treatment for PSC. Analysis of multiple cause of death files in the US between 1990 and 1998[33] shows that there was a significant decrease in mortality in women under 65 with PBC while PSC mortality remained essentially stable. In a review of United Network for Organ Sharing (UNOS) data between 1995 and 2006, Lee[34] did not find any significant change in the number of patients with PSC being listed for transplantation. Patients with PBC, however, make up an ever decreasing proportion of the transplant wait list, despite a stable incidence of PBC. This underlines UDCA's efficacy in an appropriate setting.

Summary

Further trials with UDCA are not likely to be of any positive use. PSC is an uncommon disease and opportunities to recruit patients to large scale trials are inherently limited. The Scandinavian study[8] failed to achieve its target enrollment despite involving 34 centers and 48 investigators achieving a rate of enrollment into the study of only 1 patient per investigator every 3.3 months. As current treatments for PSC are ineffective, efforts should be directed toward looking at other novel bile acids such as 24-norUDCA, currently in trial. UDCA may have a role to play in preventing colonic dysplasia, but other agents have been well researched and surely equally deserve our attention. The continued unsubstantiated faith of many in UDCA can only serve to delay us from exploring new and promising treatments for PSC.

KEY POINTS

- Trials studying the efficacy of moderate doses of UDCA (17 to 20 mg/kg/day) are inconclusive.
- High-dose UDCA (25 to 30 mg/kg/day) may be harmful particularly to patients with advanced PSC.
- Chemoprotective effect of UDCA against colonic/dysplasia and cancer has not been proven in prospective trials.
- There is no controlled evidence that UDCA protects against the development of cholagiocarcinoma.

EXPERT OPINION

Is Ursodeoxycholic Acid Useful in the Treatment of Primary Sclerosing Cholangitis? Still More Questions Than Answers

by Roger W. Chapman, MD, FRCP

How can these confusing data on the safety and efficacy of UDCA for the treatment of PSC be summarized? Whether moderate doses of UDCA slow the progression of PSC-related liver disease remains unclear and, indeed, high doses of UDCA may be harmful. However, on the basis of available data, it would be premature to write off the use of bile acids as a potential therapy for patients with PSC. As described above, retrospective data suggest that low dose UDCA (10 to 15 mg/kg per day) may have a chemoprotective role in reducing the increased prevalence of colonic neoplasia in patients with PSC.[18] Furthermore, limited evidence from observational studies suggests that UDCA may reduce the risk of cholangiocarcinoma in patients with PSC.[21]

The two sections above clearly illustrate the dilemma facing clinicians wishing to treat patients with PSC. The dilemma has resulted in a clear difference of opinion between hepatologists in North America and Europe, illustrated by the recent publication of guidelines from the European Association for the Study of the Liver (EASL)[35,36] and the American Association for Study of the Liver (AASLD).[36]

The AASLD guidelines state unequivocally that, "ursodeoxycholic acid is not indicated for the treatment of PSC." In contrast, the EASL guidelines are that "UDCA (15 to 20 mg/d) improves serum liver tests and surrogate markers of prognosis, but does not exert a proven benefit on survival. The limited data base does not yet allow a specific recommendation for the general use of UDCA in PSC." The guidelines go on to state that, "there is suggestive but limited evidence for the use of UDCA for chemoprevention of colorectal cancer (CRC) in PSC. UDCA may be particularly considered in high risk groups such as a strong family history of CRC, previous colorectal neoplasia, or longstanding extensive colitis."

What is the future of medical therapy for PSC? Novel bile acids, such as 24-norursodeoxycholic acid (norUDCA), are becoming available. NorUDCA has unique effects on biliary physiology, including the stimulation of bicarbonate-rich bile flow, which flushes injured bile ducts thereby removing toxic bile acids. NorUDCA, unlike UDCA, has been shown to have antifibrotic, anti-inflammatory, and antiproliferative effects in a mouse model of cholangitis and biliary disease.[37] Clinical studies of norUDCA in patients with cholestatic liver disease are underway.

The development of new therapies for PSC is hindered by the fact that this disease is uncommon and slowly progressive in nature. Multicenter, randomized, controlled trials are essential to evaluate survival; however, conducting such studies in PSC requires large numbers of patients and long treatment and follow-up durations. Pilot studies in PSC, therefore, remain crucial. In addition, surrogate markers of efficacy, such as standard liver function tests and liver histology, have proved to be inadequate in studies of PSC. New surrogate markers of efficacy are required and might include serum markers of fibrosis and assessment by magnetic resonance cholangio-pancreatography.

Novel bile acids and biological agents that are specifically designed to halt the progression of hepatobiliary disease offer hope for the future treatment of patients with PSC. In my opinion, high-dose UDCA (28 to 30 mg/kg/day) should no longer be used for the treatment of patients with PSC. The putative chemoprotective action of UDCA in low or moderate doses needs to be fully evaluated.

KEY POINTS

- Data on the safety and efficacy of UDCA in the treatment of patients with PSC are confusing.

- Moderate doses of UDCA (17 to 20 mg/kg/day) are safe with a trend to benefit in survival.

- High doses of UDCA (28 to 30 mg/kg/day) may be harmful and should not be used in the treatment of PSC.

- More studies are required to assess the possible chemoprotective effect of UDCA on cholangiocarcinoma and colonic cancer in patients with PSC.

References

1. Maggs JR, Chapman RW. An update on primary sclerosing cholangitis. *Curr Opin Gastroenterol.* 2008;24(3):377-383.
2. Chapman RW. High-dose ursodeoxycholic acid in the treatment of primary sclerosing cholangitis: throwing the urso out with the bathwater? *Hepatology.* 2009;50(3):671-673.
3. Lindor KD, Kowdley KV, Luketic VA, et al. High-dose ursodeoxycholic acid for the treatment of primary sclerosing cholangitis. *Hepatology.* 2009;50(3):808-814.
4. Colombo C, Crosignani A, Assaisso M, et al. Ursodeoxycholic acid therapy in cystic fibrosis-associated liver disease: a dose-response study. *Hepatology.* 1992;16(4):924-930.
5. Beuers U, Spengler U, Kruis W, et al. Ursodeoxycholic acid for treatment of primary sclerosing cholangitis: a placebo-controlled trial. *Hepatology.* 1992;16(3):707-714.
6. Batta AK, Salen G, Holubec H, Brasitus TA, Alberts D, Earnest DL. Enrichment of the more hydrophilic bile acid ursodeoxycholic acid in the fecal water-soluble fraction after feeding to rats with colon polyps. *Cancer Res.* 1998;58(8):1684-1687.
7. Lindor KD. Ursodiol for primary sclerosing cholangitis. Mayo Primary Sclerosing Cholangitis-Ursodeoxycholic Acid Study Group. *N Engl J Med.* 1997;336(10):691-695.
8. Olsson R, Boberg KM, de Muckadell OS, et al. High-dose ursodeoxycholic acid in primary sclerosing cholangitis: a 5-year multicenter, randomized, controlled study. *Gastroenterology.* 2005;129(5):1464-1472.
9. Ponsioen CY, Vrouenraets SM, Prawirodirdjo W, et al. Natural history of primary sclerosing cholangitis and prognostic value of cholangiography in a Dutch population. *Gut.* 2002;51(4):562-566.
10. Stiehl A, Walker S, Stiehl L, Rudolph G, Hofmann WJ, Theilmann L. Effect of ursodeoxycholic acid on liver and bile duct disease in primary sclerosing cholangitis. A 3-year pilot study with a placebo-controlled study period. *J Hepatol.* 1994;20(1):57-64.
11. Mitchell SA, Bansi DS, Hunt N, Von Bergmann K, Fleming KA, Chapman RW. A preliminary trial of high-dose ursodeoxycholic acid in primary sclerosing cholangitis. *Gastroenterology.* 2001;121(4):900-907.
12. Harnois DM, Angulo P, Jorgensen RA, Larusso NF, Lindor KD. High-dose ursodeoxycholic acid as a therapy for patients with primary sclerosing cholangitis. *Am J Gastroenterol.* 2001;96(5):1558-1562.
13. Okolicsanyi L, Groppo M, Floreani A, et al. Treatment of primary sclerosing cholangitis with low-dose ursodeoxycholic acid: results of a retrospective Italian multicentre survey. *Dig Liver Dis.* 2003;35(5):325-331.

14. Bergquist A, Ekbom A, Olsson R, et al. Hepatic and extrahepatic malignancies in primary sclerosing cholangitis. *J Hepatol.* 2002;36(3):321-327.

15. Martinez JD, Stratagoules ED, LaRue JM, et al. Different bile acids exhibit distinct biological effects: the tumor promoter deoxycholic acid induces apoptosis and the chemopreventive agent ursodeoxycholic acid inhibits cell proliferation. *Nutr Cancer.* 1998;31(2):111-118.

16. Broome U, Lofberg R, Lundqvist K, Veress B. Subclinical time span of inflammatory bowel disease in patients with primary sclerosing cholangitis. *Dis Colon Rectum.* 1995;38(12):1301-1305.

17. Tung BY, Emond MJ, Haggitt RC, et al. Ursodiol use is associated with lower prevalence of colonic neoplasia in patients with ulcerative colitis and primary sclerosing cholangitis. *Ann Intern Med.* 2001;134(2):89-95.

18. Pardi DS, Loftus EV, Jr., Kremers WK, Keach J, Lindor KD. Ursodeoxycholic acid as a chemopreventive agent in patients with ulcerative colitis and primary sclerosing cholangitis. *Gastroenterology.* 2003;124(4):889-893.

19. Wolf JM, Rybicki LA, Lashner BA. The impact of ursodeoxycholic acid on cancer, dysplasia and mortality in ulcerative colitis patients with primary sclerosing cholangitis. *Aliment Pharmacol Ther.* 2005;22(9):783-788.

20. Boberg KM, Bergquist A, Mitchell S, et al. Cholangiocarcinoma in primary sclerosing cholangitis: risk factors and clinical presentation. *Scand J Gastroenterol.* 2002;37(10):1205-1211.

21. Brandsaeter B, Isoniemi H, Broome U, et al. Liver transplantation for primary sclerosing cholangitis; predictors and consequences of hepatobiliary malignancy. *J Hepatol.* 2004;40(5):815-822.

22. Cullen SN, Rust C, Fleming K, Edwards C, Beuers U, Chapman RW. High dose ursodeoxycholic acid for the treatment of primary sclerosing cholangitis is safe and effective. *J Hepatol.* 2008;48(5):792-800.

23. Rost D, Rudolph G, Kloeters-Plachky P, Stiehl A. Effect of high-dose ursodeoxycholic acid on its biliary enrichment in primary sclerosing cholangitis. *Hepatology.* 2004;40(3):693-698.

24. Sinakos E, Marschall HU, Kowdley KV, Befeler A, Keach J, Lindor K. Bile acid changes after high-dose ursodeoxycholic acid treatment in primary sclerosing cholangitis: relation to disease progression. *Hepatology.* 2010;52(1):197-203.

25. Shi J, Wu C, Lin Y, Chen YX, Zhu L, Xie WF. Long-term effects of mid-dose ursodeoxycholic acid in primary biliary cirrhosis: a meta-analysis of randomized controlled trials. *Am J Gastroenterol.* 2006;101(7):1529-1538.

26. Chazouilleres O, Poupon R, Capron JP, et al. Ursodeoxycholic acid for primary sclerosing cholangitis. *J Hepatol.* 1990;11(1):120-123.

27. O'Brien CB, Senior JR, Arora-Mirchandani R, Batta AK, Salen G. Ursodeoxycholic acid for the treatment of primary sclerosing cholangitis: a 30-month pilot study. *Hepatology.* 1991;14(5):838-847.

28. Poupon RE, Balkau B, Eschwege E, Poupon R. A multicenter, controlled trial of ursodiol for the treatment of primary biliary cirrhosis. UDCA-PBC Study Group. *N Engl J Med.* 1991;324(22):1548-1554.

29. Olsson R, Hagerstrand I, Broome U, et al. Sampling variability of percutaneous liver biopsy in primary sclerosing cholangitis. *J Clin Pathol.* 1995;48(10):933-935.

30. Shi J, Li Z, Zeng X, Lin Y, Xie WF. Ursodeoxycholic acid in primary sclerosing cholangitis: meta-analysis of randomized controlled trials. *Hepatol Res.* 2009;39(9):865-873.

31. Charatcharoenwitthaya P, Angulo P, Enders FB, Lindor KD. Impact of inflammatory bowel disease and ursodeoxycholic acid therapy on small-duct primary sclerosing cholangitis. *Hepatology.* 2008;47(1):133-142.

32. Shetty K, Rybicki L, Brzezinski A, Carey WD, Lashner BA. The risk for cancer or dysplasia in ulcerative colitis patients with primary sclerosing cholangitis. *Am J Gastroenterol.* 1999;94(6):1643-1649.

33. Mendes FD, Kim WR, Pedersen R, Therneau T, Lindor KD. Mortality attributable to cholestatic liver disease in the United States. *Hepatology.* 2008;47(4):1241-1247.

34. Lee J, Belanger A, Doucette JT, Stanca C, Friedman S, Bach N. Transplantation trends in primary biliary cirrhosis. *Clin Gastroenterol Hepatol.* 2007;5(11):1313-1315.

35. EASL Clinical Practice Guidelines: management of cholestatic liver diseases. *J Hepatol.* 2009;51(2):237-267.

36. Chapman R, Fevery J, Kalloo A, et al. Diagnosis and management of primary sclerosing cholangitis. *Hepatology.* 2010;51(2):660-678.

37. Fickert P, Wagner M, Marschall HU, et al. 24-norUrsodeoxycholic acid is superior to ursodeoxycholic acid in the treatment of sclerosing cholangitis in Mdr2 (Abcb4) knockout mice. *Gastroenterology.* 2006;130(2):465-481.

CHAPTER 15

Annual Screening of Primary Sclerosing Cholangitis Patients for Cholangiocarcinoma With Magnetic Resonance Cholangiopancreatography and CA 19-9?

Boris Blechacz, MD, PhD; Nataliya Razumilava, MD; and Gregory J. Gores, MD

With a 10% lifetime risk of developing cholangiocarcinoma, patients with primary sclerosing cholangitis (PSC) would seem a natural group with which to implement cancer surveillance. Unfortunately, no current guidelines recommend annual surveillance, in part because of the lack of good prospective data. Does this mean, however, that we should not screen our PSC patients? The two sides of active surveillance, for and against, are discussed in the following chapter.

Jensen D.
*Controversies in Hepatology: The Experts Analyze Both
Sides (pp 145-152)*
© 2011 SLACK Incorporated

POINT

Cholangiocarcinoma Surveillance Is the Key for Cure in Primary Sclerosing Cholangitis Patients With This Otherwise Lethal Malignancy

by Boris Blechacz, MD, PhD

Cholangiocarcinoma in Primary Sclerosing Cholangitis: Risk, Treatment, and Prognosis

Primary sclerosing cholangitis (PSC) is the most established risk factor for the development of cholangiocarcinoma (CCA). Up to 10% of PSC patients will develop CCA.[1,2] Certain subgroups of PSC patients are at a 25-fold increased risk for the development of CCA.[2] Patients diagnosed with CCA have a median survival of 4.6 months.[3] Conventional antineoplastic agents have minimal efficacy on long-term survival. The only potentially curative treatments are surgical, including resection or liver transplantation with 5-year survival rates of up to 63% and 79%, respectively.[4,5] However, the indications for these surgical approaches are highly limited and depend on tumor location, extent, size, and the absence of metastatic disease. Outcomes of resection for CCA highly depend on tumor stage and type of resection. R0 resection (curative resection) achieved 72% 1-year survival versus 27% and 31%, respectively, with R1 (microscopic residual disease) and R2 (macroscopic residual disease) resection, respectively.[6] Using the fifth and sixth edition of the Union Internationale Contre Cancer (UICC) staging classification for intrahepatic CCA, it was shown on multivariate analysis that stages I and II had significantly better outcomes than more advanced stages.[6] Similarly for perihilar CCA undergoing liver transplantation, it was shown that high CA 19-9 serum concentrations as well as visible masses on axial imaging have a negative impact on outcomes.[5] Hence, early detection of CCA is key for a potentially curative therapeutic approach.

How Good Are CA 19-9 and Magnetic Resonance Cholangiopancreatography for the Diagnosis of Cholangiocarcinoma?

CCA are difficult to diagnose and frequently require a combination of different modalities as well as expertise in their interpretation. However, serum analysis for CA 19-9 and MRI/magnetic resonance cholangiopancreatography (MRCP) are readily available in most centers. In PSC, CA 19-9 has a sensitivity of 78.6% and a specificity of 98.5% at a cut-off serum concentration of equal or more than 129 U/mL. A change of CA 19-9 serum concentration of 67.3% over time in these patients has a sensitivity and specificity of 90% and 98%.[7] MRCP is obtained in conjunction with MRI. MRI/MRCP has a reported diagnostic accuracy of up to 94%, sensitivity and specificity of up to 100% and 94%, and a positive and negative predictive value of up to 96% and 100%.[8,9] The accuracy for prediction of tumor extent is 85% to 89%, for vascular involvement 86% to 96%, and for lymph node metastases 74%.[10] Patients with PSC are especially challenging due to the development of strictures in the natural history of this chronic inflammatory biliary disease. MRCP is less invasive than endoscopic retrograde cholangiopancreatography (ERCP) and has a comparable sensitivity, specificity, and accuracy for differentiation of malignant from benign causes of biliary stricture of 81%, 70%, and 76%.[11]

Is Cost an Issue?

Cost-effectiveness is a frequent argument against surveillance for diseases in at-risk populations. However, the incidence of PSC as well as CCA has significantly increased within the last 2 decades.[12,13] The impact of this disease on the prognosis is dismal, with survival of less than 24 months after diagnosis.[1] The average age for the diagnosis of PSC is reported to be between 40 to 47 years and for CCA 50 years.[1,14] Hence, the impact of CCA in PSC is devastating for the individual patient and his or her family, and economically for society at large given the young age of these patients (loss of economic productivity due to premature death). The current Medicare fee for CA 19-9 is $30 and for MRCP $796. With the increase in disease prevalence, the diagnostic accuracy—in particular the positive predictive value of diagnostic tests—will increase. Beyond discussion of costs and financial concerns, the moral obligation of physicians toward their patients should not be forgotten. Many PSC patients have a very good understanding of their disease and are aware of their risk for the development of this malignancy. Especially after the diagnosis has been made, many patients are distressed about the possibility of developing a highly lethal malignancy and appreciate careful and thorough surveillance.

Summary

CCA is a lethal disease for which PSC patients are at high risk. Its prognosis is dismal. Surgical treatment approaches are the only chance for cure. However, localized disease is a requirement for surgical therapy. Analysis of serum CA 19-9 concentration and MRI/MRCP are noninvasive, readily available, and relatively inexpensive methods that have been shown to identify and stage this malignancy with good diagnostic accuracy. Their accuracy in predicting tumor location, extent, and resectability have been shown and provide these patients the opportunity for potentially curative treatments in this otherwise lethal disease. Questions that remain include optimal surveillance intervals and impact on the combination of CA 19-9 combined with MRI/MRCP on the diagnostic accuracy for CCA surveillance in PSC.

KEY POINTS

- Early detection of cholangiocarcinoma offers the only realistic chance for curative intervention.
- For structured imaging of the biliary tree, MRI/MRCP can be performed safely and with diagnostic accuracy.
- The physician has an obligation to maintain a patient's health with the best surveillance tools available, even if unproven.

COUNTERPOINT

Evidence Is Lacking to Implement Cholangiocarcinoma Surveillance in Primary Sclerosing Cholangitis Patients

by Nataliya Razumilava, MD

Are We Ready for Cholangiocarcinoma Surveillance in Patients With Primary Sclerosing Cholangitis?

In the absence of data, medical decision making can be a confusing process with which every physician must grapple to provide the best care for his or her individual patient. In this context, the increased rate of CCA development in PSC patients leads physicians to consider surveillance for CCA in PSC patients, despite the absence of compelling data.

Per definition, surveillance represents a strategy for disease detection in an asymptomatic at-risk population, with an ultimate goal to detect and treat disease at an earlier stage, resulting in improved outcomes (Figure 15-1). Important components of a successful surveillance strategy include identifying the population at risk; available, accessible, and acceptable surveillance modalities; surveillance tools with high sensitivity and specificity; available and agreed-upon treatment options; cost effectiveness of the process; and improved outcomes as a result of early detection. Unfortunately, none of these components are firmly established regarding surveillance of PSC patients with CCA.

Do We Have an Identifiable Population at Risk?

PSC represents a major risk factor for CCA with reported prevalence ranging from 5% to 10% depending on the studied population. However, it is likely that only a subset of PSC patients are at high risk and would benefit from aggressive surveillance strategies. Unlike colorectal cancer risk in ulcerative colitis, a correlation between CCA and duration of PSC has not been demonstrated; in fact, an inverse correlation has been suggested.[15] Unfortunately, although many factors have been reported to increase the risk for CCA in PSC patients (elevated bilirubin, polymorphism of the NKG2D gene, presence of colorectal cancer or dysplasia in patients with ulcerative colitis, the duration of inflammatory bowel disease, proctocolectomy, variceal bleeding, smoking, alcohol use, and older age at PSC diagnosis), these studies have not been uniformly replicated or verified.[16-19] Thus, we still have inadequate information to identify the subset of patients at higher risk for developing CCA.

What Are the Surveillance Modalities and Their Performance Characteristics?

Physicians want surveillance tests to have high sensitivity, which allows for disease detection with a low rate of false negatives, and high specificity, which reduces false positives. However,

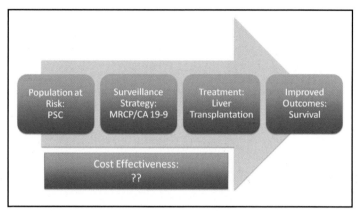

Figure 15-1. Decision-making analysis of disease surveillance.

combined use of MRCP and CA 19-9 testing with a cutoff value for CA 19-9 of ≥20 U/mL, with either test being positive, yields a sensitivity of 100% but a specificity of only 38%. Choosing a cutoff value of ≥129 U/mL improves the specificity, but it also decreases the sensitivity.[20]

One might consider ERCP as an alternative surveillance strategy that permits specimen acquisition for cytology and fluorescence in situ hybridization (FISH) analysis. However, no information is available to support this approach. Also, ERCP is fraught with complications in this patient group, making it undesirable as a surveillance test.[21] Thus, we do not have acceptable tests to diagnose early CCA in this disease population.

What Are the Limitations of Surveillance Modalities?

The large number of potential false-positive results with MRI and serum CA 19-9 testing will require further investigation. Most likely, a concern will prompt an ERCP or phenylthiocarbamide (PTC) with sampling for cytopathologic evaluation, including FISH analysis where available, and additional cross-sectional imaging studies. Thus, many patients who do not have cancer will undergo unnecessary testing with added anxiety, procedural complications, and significant expenses. Some of these patients will develop cholangitis and pancreatitis, which will result in iatrogenic harm.

What Are the Treatment Options Available for Cholangiocarcinoma?

It is possible that survival from time of diagnosis will increase in patients who undergo surveillance as a consequence of lead time bias, rather than increase in overall life span. Thus, patients may spend more time anxiously knowing about their diagnosis but not derive a survival benefit. Tumors detected by surveillance may have a different natural history compared to tumors with more aggressive symptomatic presentation. This will lead to length/time bias, as survival will be longer but not due to earlier detection. Furthermore, there is no standardized therapeutic approach. Surgical resection as a definitive treatment can only be offered to a limited number of patients with an early intra- or extrahepatic disease with reasonably preserved liver function to avoid decompensation. Even in this highly selected population, surgery is associated with a 3-year survival rate <20%. Liver transplantation has been proposed as a solution to improve outcomes in perihilar tumors. However, when performed alone, it is associated with an unacceptably high tumor recurrence rate. The best outcomes with 5-year survival above

70% have been demonstrated in highly selective patients with early stage perihilar CCA who undergo neoadjuvant chemotherapy followed by liver transplantation.[5] Thus, there is a therapeutic option for early stage CCA in PSC patients, but its cost-effectiveness is unclear.

Is Surveillance Cost-Effective?

Proposed surveillance modalities for CCA and resulting increase in testing are costly. No study has evaluated the cost-effectiveness of different surveillance approaches with ratio calculation of cost per year of life saved. Moreover, quality-adjusted life year, another important index in a decision analysis, is often based on individual values and beliefs and cannot be applied universally.

Summary

Making a decision about the best surveillance strategy for our patients who suffer from a progressive and potentially deadly disease is very challenging and requires a systematic approach. Imperfect surveillance characteristics, lack of standardized approach to work-up, recall, and treatment indicate that we cannot advocate surveillance in this patient population; we simply do not have sufficient evidence to justify such a recommendation.

KEY POINTS

- It is not possible to identify the high-risk population.
- Surveillance will optimally require tissue or cytologic sampling, which is too invasive and risky by ERCP to justify.
- Cost-effectiveness of interval CA 19-9 plus MRI based surveillance is unknown.

EXPERT OPINION

A Pragmatic Approach Regarding Cholangiocarcinoma Surveillance in Primary Sclerosing Cholangitis Patients

by Gregory J. Gores, MD

The issue of surveillance for CCA in PSC patients was recently addressed by the practice guidelines committees of the American Association for the Study of Liver Diseases (AASLD)[22] and the European Association for the Study of Liver Diseases (EASL).[23] The AASLD guidelines simply stated that "inadequate information exists regarding the utility of screening for CCA in PSC; in the absence of evidence based information, many clinicians screen patients with an imaging study plus a CA 19-9 at annual intervals." The EASL guidelines gave the recommendation that "there is, at present, no biochemical marker or imaging modality which can be recommended for early detection of cholangiocarcinoma. ERCP with brush cytology (and/or biopsy) sampling should be carried out when clinically indicated." These guidelines were so written because there are no high quality studies to justify surveillance from an evidence-based perspective. Indeed, I wrote this section of the AASLD guidelines, although I practice differently.

As both Drs. Blechacz and Razumilava highlight, the individual patient is seeking our care and guidance to improve his or her quality of life and longevity. They want to avail themselves of our expertise, experience, and judgment and trust that we will personalize their care and not merely practice within the confines of practice guidelines. The absence of high quality information also does not imply that surveillance is wrong, only that the proper studies have not been performed. In this regard, like my colleague Dr. Keith Lindor from the Mayo Clinic located in Rochester, MN, we do advocate for and practice surveillance for hepatobiliary malignancy in PSC patients, but with rather different approaches. I have had the experience of a rising serum CA 19-9 determination herald the presence of an unexpected CCA. Therefore, I include this serum test in my management panel ("hot button orders") in the care of PSC patients. PSC is a structural disease of the biliary tract and, therefore, I also prefer to obtain an MRI along with an MRCP on annual basis. I reserve ERCP plus brush cytology (ie, conventional cytology and FISH) for those patients with progressive strictures on an MRCP, jaundice, history of cholangitis, or a CA 19-9 that is rising and above 100 U/mL. Dr. Lindor prefers to obtain an ultrasound to examine for progressive segmental bile duct dilatation and enhanced bile duct wall thickness. He also reserves ERCP examinations for clinical indications. Our pro-surveillance posture is greatly influenced by the Mayo Clinic protocol employing neoadjuvant chemoradiation followed by orthotopic liver transplantation as definitive therapy for early CCA in the setting of PSC.[5] Long-term outcome data for PSC patients with early CCA are virtually identical to those for patients undergoing liver transplantation for cirrhosis. Thus, we can potentially cure early stage CCA in PSC patients with this approach, providing a rationale for making an early diagnosis. Thus, from my perspective, we have a population of patients at risk for the development of CCA (ie, PSC patients), we have adequate screening modalities, and a potential life-saving treatment option for those patients identified during surveillance testing. The cost-effectiveness of this approach is unclear and has not been modeled; an erstwhile endeavor albeit fraught with several assumptions. Although randomized controlled trials would be useful to address this issue, it is unlikely any will ever be conducted. First, the disease has a low incidence and few centers have large populations of PSC patients. Second, the study would be confounded (ie, contamination of the nonimaging arm) by the use of imaging studies prompted by changes in clinical status. Third, not all patients and centers are in a position to avail themselves of the chemoradiation neoadjuvant protocol followed by liver transplantation to treat patients with early stage CCA. Therefore, surveillance fails to improve clinical outcome for such patients and their centers. Likely, those of us who practice surveillance will need to retrospectively examine our practices and ascertain their benefit over time. In the interim, I suggest we do perform surveillance as previously described.

References

1. Blechacz B, Gores GJ. Cholangiocarcinoma: advances in pathogenesis, diagnosis, and treatment. *Hepatology*. 2008;48(1):308-321.
2. Burak K, Angulo P, Pasha TM, et al. Incidence and risk factors for cholangiocarcinoma in primary sclerosing cholangitis. *Am J Gastroenterol*. 2004;99(3):523-526.
3. Key C, Meisner ALW. Cancers of the liver and biliary tract. In: Ries LAG, Young JL, Keel GE, (eds). *SEER Survival Monograph, Cancer Survival Among Adults: US SEER Program, 1988-2001, Patient and Tumor Characteristics*. Bethesda, MD: National Cancer Institute; 2007.
4. Blechacz BR, Gores GJ. Cholangiocarcinoma. *Clin Liver Dis*. 2008;12(1):131-150.
5. Rosen CB, Heimbach JK, Gores GJ. Liver transplantation for cholangiocarcinoma. *Transpl Int*. 2010;23(7):692-697.
6. Jonas S, Thelen A, Benckert C, et al. Extended liver resection for intrahepatic cholangiocarcinoma: a comparison of the prognostic accuracy of the fifth and sixth editions of the TNM classification. *Ann Surg*. 2009;249(2):303-309.
7. Levy C, Lymp J, Angulo P, et al. The value of serum CA 19-9 in predicting cholangiocarcinomas in patients with primary sclerosing cholangitis. *Dig Dis Sci*. 2005;50(9):1734-1740.
8. Kim JY, Kim MH, Lee TY, et al. Clinical role of 18F-FDG PET-CT in suspected and potentially operable cholangiocarcinoma: a prospective study compared with conventional imaging. *Am J Gastroenterol*. 2008;103(5):1145-1151.
9. Cui XY, Chen HW. Role of diffusion-weighted magnetic resonance imaging in the diagnosis of extrahepatic cholangiocarcinoma. *World J Gastroenterol*. 2010;16(25):3196-3201.
10. Park HS, Lee JM, Choi JY, et al. Preoperative evaluation of bile duct cancer: MRI combined with MR cholangiopancreatography versus MDCT with direct cholangiography. *Am J Roentgenol*. 2008;190(2):396-405.
11. Park MS, Kim TK, Kim KW, et al. Differentiation of extrahepatic bile duct cholangiocarcinoma from benign stricture: findings at MRCP versus ERCP. *Radiology*. 2004;233(1):234-240.
12. Everhart JE, Ruhl CE. Burden of digestive diseases in the United States Part III: liver, biliary tract, and pancreas. *Gastroenterology*. 2009;136(4):1134-1144.
13. Lindkvist B, Benito de Valle M, Gullberg B, Bjornsson E. Incidence and prevalence of primary sclerosing cholangitis in a defined adult population in Sweden. *Hepatology*. 2010;52(2):571-577.
14. Shorbagi A, Bayraktar Y. Primary sclerosing cholangitis--what is the difference between east and west? *World J Gastroenterol*. 2008;14(25):3974-3981.
15. Lazaridis KN, Gores GJ. Primary sclerosing cholangitis and cholangiocarcinoma. *Semin Liver Dis*. 2006;26(1):42-51.
16. Melum E, Karlsen TH, Schrumpf E, et al. Cholangiocarcinoma in primary sclerosing cholangitis is associated with NKG2D polymorphisms. *Hepatology*. 2008;47(1):90-96.
17. Bergquist A, Ekbom A, Olsson R, et al. Hepatic and extrahepatic malignancies in primary sclerosing cholangitis. *J Hepatol*. 2002;36(3):321-327.
18. Boberg KM, Bergquist A, Mitchell S, et al. Cholangiocarcinoma in primary sclerosing cholangitis: risk factors and clinical presentation. *Scand J Gastroenterol*. 2002;37(10):1205-1211.
19. Broome U, Lofberg R, Veress B, Eriksson LS. Primary sclerosing cholangitis and ulcerative colitis: evidence for increased neoplastic potential. *Hepatology*. 1995;22(5):1404-1408.
20. Charatcharoenwitthaya P, Enders FB, Halling KC, et al. Utility of serum tumor markers, imaging, and biliary cytology for detecting cholangiocarcinoma in primary sclerosing cholangitis. *Hepatology*. 2008;48(4):1106-1117.
21. Bangarulingam SY, Gossard AA, Petersen BT, et al. Complications of endoscopic retrograde cholangiopancreatography in primary sclerosing cholangitis. *Am J Gastroenterol*. 2009;104(4):855-860.
22. Chapman R, Fevery J, Kalloo A, et al. Diagnosis and management of primary sclerosing cholangitis. American Association for the Study of Liver Disease. *Hepatology*. 2010;51(2):660-678.
23. EASL Clinical Practice Guidelines: management of cholestatic liver diseases. European Association for the Study of the Liver. *J Hepatol*. 2009;51(2):237-267.

CHAPTER 16

LACTULOSE OR RIFAXIMIN AS FIRST-LINE THERAPY FOR HEPATIC ENCEPHALOPATHY?

Tarek I. Abu-Rajab Tamimi, MD; Thomas A. Brown, MD; and Kevin D. Mullen, MD

The primary issue regarding whether lactulose or rifaximin should be first-line of therapy for treatment of hepatic encephalopathy hinges on efficiency and cost.

POINT

Lactulose as First-Line Therapy for Hepatic Encephalopathy

by Tarek I. Abu-Rajab Tamimi, MD

Lactulose has been an approved therapy for hepatic encephalopathy (HE) since 1977. Johannes Bircher first clinically introduced it in a report of a series of cases in 1971.[1] Prior to that, neomycin was mainly used for the treatment of HE. However, long-term use of neomycin is associated with nephrotoxicity and ototoxicity. Therefore, lactulose was gradually adopted as a mainstay of therapy for HE.

Lactulose is a synthetic, nonabsorbable disaccharide, which allows it to reach to the colon and exert its effects there. The colonic flora metabolizes lactulose to short chain fatty acids, which lowers the colonic pH. This acidic environment traps ammonia in the colon in the form of $NH4+$, thereby reducing plasma ammonia concentrations. Other mechanisms of action include increased incorporation of ammonia by bacteria for synthesis of nitrogenous compounds, modification of colonic flora resulting in displacement of urease-containing bacteria with *Lactobacillus*, in addition to the mere laxative effect, which reduces the contact time to absorb ammonia. Therefore, lactulose reduces ammonia generation and absorption from the gut.

Jensen D.
Controversies in Hepatology: The Experts Analyze Both Sides (pp 153-158)
© 2011 SLACK Incorporated

Lactulose was considered to be as effective as neomycin in the treatment of HE.[2,3] Since then, there has been extensive clinical experience supporting the efficacy of lactulose. In a systematic review, Als-Nielsen et al found that nonabsorbable disaccharides were more effective than placebo or no intervention in treating HE in 6 trials.[4] Moreover, a study conducted by Prasad et al found that treatment with lactulose improved both cognitive function and health-related quality of life in patients with minimal HE.[5] Even though the latter study was not placebo-controlled, this mild form of HE has allowed placebo-controlled trials, which added greatly to the credibility of lactulose. Sharma et al[6] found that lactulose significantly decreased the recurrence of overt HE compared to placebo (20% versus 47% over a 14 month follow-up period). However, readmission rates due to causes other than HE and mortality in both groups were similar. One major advantage of lactulose is its relatively low cost. Lactulose dose is best titrated to induce 2 to 3 loose bowel movements daily.

On the other hand, there is a lack of sufficiently sized, well-designed, placebo-controlled studies to prove the efficacy of lactulose in treating HE. In the same systematic review stated above,[4] when only trials of high methodological quality were considered (2 trials), they found that there was no significant effect of nonabsorbable disaccharides on improvement of HE. They also found that nonabsorbable disaccharides appeared to be less effective than antibiotics in improving HE. In the majority of cases of overt HE, a precipitating factor or factors can be identified. The role of these precipitating factors has not been properly accounted for in many treatment trials for HE. This raised the suspicion that identifying and treating these precipitating factors in the setting of overt HE may be more important than the therapeutic effect of lactulose or other medications targeting HE.[7] Another limitation to the lactulose trials is that truly blinded studies are difficult to conduct because of the laxative effect of lactulose. It has been postulated that any laxative may have an effect in managing HE by decreasing the ammonia absorption time from the gut. So when a laxative agent was added to the comparator or placebo to match the diarrhea induced by lactulose, the comparison was most probably inaccurate. The most common complaints associated with lactulose include its excessive sweet taste, abdominal cramping, flatulence, and diarrhea. Overdosing lactulose may lead to excessive diarrhea with dehydration and electrolyte abnormalities, which may worsen the patient's mental status.

Limitations to the lactulose treatment trials may be due to the following:

- Confounding effect of associated precipitating factors for HE and their treatment.
- Inability to conduct truly blinded studies due to the laxative effect of lactulose.
- Excessive sweet taste, abdominal cramping, flatulence, and diarrhea with possible dehydration and electrolyte abnormalities.

KEY POINTS

- There is extensive data indicating the potential mechanisms of action for decreasing serum ammonia concentration.
- Clinical experience supports the efficacy of lactulose.
- Improvement of minimal HE has been found.
- There is decreased recurrence rate of overt HE.
- No severe adverse events have been found.
- This is a low cost option.
- There is a lack of sufficiently sized, well-designed, placebo-controlled studies.

COUNTERPOINT

Rifaximin as First-Line Therapy for Hepatic Encephalopathy

by Thomas A. Brown, MD

Rifaximin should be a first-line treatment used at the initial appearance of overt hepatic encephalopathy (HE) in the setting of cirrhosis (ie, type C overt HE). Head-to-head comparisons have proven similar efficacies between rifaximin and lactulose/lactitol as well as effectiveness of rifaximin when used for lactulose nonresponders, yet rifaximin is better tolerated and associated with decreased costs when considering both shortening hospital admissions and preventing future admissions.[8-12]

Rifaximin is considerably more expensive than lactulose as a prescription, yet one must consider the natural history of HE to understand the reasoning behind the cost benefit of rifaximin. Once overt HE first appears in the setting of cirrhosis, it typically becomes a relapsing/remitting disorder. It is recommended that most patients who develop symptoms of overt HE be admitted to the hospital to rapidly diagnose and correct any precipitating factors such as infection, bleeding, and dehydration as well as to prevent deepening of the HE. Each hospital admission for HE typically lasts several days and often a patient is placed in the intensive care unit initially if he or she cannot adequately protect his or her airway as is seen in grade 4 or sometimes grade 3. Leevy et al showed rifaximin is associated with a significantly shortened length of stay when compared to lactulose (2.5 days versus 7.3 days, respectively).[11] Neff et al showed similarly significant results (3.5 days versus 5 days).[9] A cycle of repeated admissions and discharges develops until either the time of death or liver transplantation. Preventing future admissions considerably decreases the costs associated with HE. Neff et al also calculated that the cost per patient per year with a history of HE on rifaximin (original 400 mg TID dosing) was significantly less than a patient on lactulose when factoring in the hospital costs ($7958 per patient per year versus $13,285 per patient per year).[9] In the important study by Bass et al, rifaximin (with concurrent lactulose in 91% of patients) reduced repeated hospitalizations by 50% compared to placebo and lactulose.[12] The number needed to treat with rifaximin to prevent an admission in 6 months was 9.

Sobering data from Bsutamante et al showed a 42% 1-year survival probability and 23% 3-year survival probability.[13] Thus, when considering initial treatments for HE, the medications will likely not be given for as long a period of time as compared to treating gastroesophageal reflux disease or diabetes mellitus. It is unknown whether rifaximin improves survival when used after the first episode of overt HE.

Recurrent bouts of HE result in a worsened quality of life, loss of autonomy, increased caregiver demands, and often loss of gainful employment. Thus, preventing future bouts of HE is crucial to keeping a patient independent and at home. According to Bass et al, rifaximin reduced the number of episodes of overt HE by 58%.[12] The number needed to treat to prevent one episode of HE in 6 months was 4.

While lactulose is notorious for causing diarrhea, abdominal cramping, bloating, flatulence, and at times nausea, the addition of rifaximin does not increase any of these side effects significantly.[12] The concern for *Clostridium difficile* by rifaximin is warranted because rifaximin is a nonabsorbable antibiotic likely to alter intestinal flora. This has not proven to be a significant problem. Rifaximin affects small intestinal bacteria more so than colonic bacteria.[14] Of 140 patients,

2 developed *C. difficile* infection while 0 of 159 treated with lactulose and placebo developed it.[12] Both of those patients had also been on multiple courses of other antibiotic therapy over numerous hospital admissions.

The relative ease of use of rifaximin (one 550 mg tablet po BID) as compared to titrating lactulose to achieve 2 to 3 soft bowel movements provides yet another advantage to rifaximin. Explaining the notion of adjusting lactulose's dose and frequency to a patient and his or her family takes considerable time and often needs to be repeated on subsequent office visits. Compliance is likely to be higher with rifaximin as patients are generally more accustomed to taking pills routinely for longer periods of time for prevention of a disorder and not just on an as-needed basis as often happens with lactulose. Finally, the sweet taste of lactulose is another deterrent to routine long-term ingestion that rifaximin bypasses.

Nonetheless, rifaximin has its drawbacks. It does not prevent 100% of relapses of HE. Also it does not rapidly resolve overt HE within a matter of seconds to minutes. While not yet investigated, rifaximin will likely have minimal to no effect on the encephalopathy seen in cases of acute liver failure (type A overt HE). It is unknown what effects rifaximin will have on the subtle condition of minimal HE.

Since one of the largest, most convincing studies to date consisted mostly of patients taking both lactulose and rifaximin,[12] it is conservative to say that rifaximin should be included in first-line therapy along with lactulose and correcting precipitating factors until larger, long-term head-to-head data of lactulose versus rifaximin are available. Should a patient develop intolerance or no response to lactulose, rifaximin should be considered as the sole agent.

KEY POINTS

- Reduction in recurrent bouts of HE by 58%.
- Reduction in hospitalizations for HE by 50%.
- Higher cost as a prescription compared to lactulose but is more cost effective when factoring in cost of hospitalizations.
- Improved tolerability.

EXPERT OPINION

First-Line Treatment of Hepatic Encephalopathy: Even More Data Needed?

by Kevin D. Mullen, MD

The therapeutic approach to the management of HE did not change much for 30 years. The primary reason for this was the early adoption of lactulose as the therapeutic agent to treat all cases of overt HE. Despite the knowledge that precipitating factor correction was the key to reversing HE in the majority of patients, lactulose quickly got all the credit for "waking up" patients from hepatic coma. Soon after it began to be considered unethical to withhold lactulose from patients with overt HE. It was then that the opportunity to finally do properly powered placebo-controlled trials with lactulose was lost. Paradoxically, as lactulose was being considered essential for HE treatment, there was a widespread overdosing of lactulose, causing at times dehydration and electrolyte disturbances.

There is no question that lactulose has efficacy in the treatment of overt HE. The administration of lactulose to a patient with overt HE and no precipitating factors is associated with recovery from what is called spontaneous HE. The major problem is that this effect was not rigorously compared to placebo and never compared to standard laxatives. In essence, lactulose was primarily compared to neomycin and other antibiotics and became widely used because of its lack of toxicity compared to neomycin. As already mentioned, we had the superimposed effects of variable correction of precipitating factors. In some studies, the comparator treatment had a laxative added to it (eg, sorbitol) to match the diarrhea induced by lactulose. This may have obscured the efficiency of lactulose. Only one study has shown a superiority of lactulose to placebo when equal bowel evacuations were applied to both arms of the study.[15] This study was an evaluation of lactulose compared to tap water enemas.

As stated earlier in the lactulose discussion, many mechanisms have been identified that reduce intestinal flora production and subsequent absorption of ammonia with lactulose. It is indeed mechanistically difficult to envisage standard type laxatives having effects on bowel flora in this fashion. So in addition to promoting evacuation of stools, lactulose may have multiple mechanisms for ultimately reducing blood ammonia. On that point I will leave lactulose.

Rifaximin, because of concerns about the ethics of not giving lactulose to patients with overt HE, has not had a pure placebo versus active drug trial. Instead patients having documented recurrent bouts of overt HE—despite 91% being already on lactulose—were randomized to receive 550 mg po BID of rifaximin or an identical placebo. The 58% reduction in bouts of overt HE with rifaximin is obviously very striking, yet the impact of the concurrent dose-controlled lactulose on the outcome is difficult to gauge. It is important to note that the participants had 1, 2, or more prior bouts of overt HE despite lactulose. If the trial participants could have had their lactulose withdrawn during the open phase follow-up, we would have an estimate of the contribution of rifaximin versus lactulose to maintenance of remission. One additional issue as the time of follow-up gets into years is that liver function may be worsening. A point may eventually be reached where prevention of bouts of overt HE may not be successful any longer.

Rifaximin may become first-line therapy for HE in all its manifestations and severity in the future. In the meantime, its reduction in hospitalizations (50%) to a significant extent justifies its considerable cost. Whether it will be cost-effective in the management of minimal HE remains to be established but appears to be a reasonable probability. Finally, it will be apparent in the near future whether rifaximin will be effective as initial treatment to patients presenting with overt episodes of HE in addition to the treatment of precipitating factors. If this is demonstrated, then rifaximin will become the first-line therapy for all forms of HE.

References

1. Bircher J, Haemmerli UP, Scollo-Lavizzari G, et al. Treatment of chronic portal-systemic encephalopathy with lactulose. Report of six patients and review of the literature. *Am J Med.* 1971;51(2):148-159.
2. Conn HO, Leevy CM, Vlahcevic ZR, et al. Comparison of lactulose and neomycin in the treatment of chronic portal-systemic encephalopathy. A double blind controlled trial. *Gastroenterology.* 1977;72(1):573-583.
3. Atterbury CE, Maddrey WC, Conn HO. Neomycin-sorbitol and lactulose in the treatment of acute portal-systemic encephalopathy. A controlled, double-blind clinical trial. *Am J Dig Dis.* 1978;23(5):398-406.
4. Als-Nielsen B, Gluud LL, Gluud C. Nonabsorbable disaccharides for hepatic encephalopathy. *Cochrane Database Syst Rev.* 2004;(2):CD003044.
5. Prasad S, Dhiman RK, Duseja A, et al. Lactulose improves cognitive functions and health-related quality of life in patients with cirrhosis who have minimal hepatic encephalopathy. *Hepatology.* 2007;45(3):549-559.
6. Sharma BC, Sharma P, Agrawal A, et al. Secondary prophylaxis of hepatic encephalopathy: an open-label randomized controlled trial of lactulose versus placebo. *Gastroenterology.* 2009;137(3):885-891.
7. Strauss E, Tramote R, Silva EP, et al. Double-blind randomized clinical trial comparing neomycin and placebo in the treatment of exogenous hepatic encephalopathy. *Hepatogastroenterology.* 1992;39(6):542-545.
8. Mas A, Rodes J, Sunyer L, et al. Comparison of rifaximin and lactitol in the treatment of acute hepatic encephalopathy: results of a randomized, double-blind, double-dummy, controlled clinical trial. *J Hepatol.* 2003;38(1):52-58.
9. Neff GW, Kemmer N, Zacharias VC, et al. Analysis of hospitalizations comparing rifaximin versus lactulose in the management of hepatic encephalopathy. *Transpl Proceedings.* 2006;38(1):3552-3555.
10. Sama C, Morselli-Labate AM, Pinata P, et al. Clinical effects of rifaximin in patients with hepatic encephalopathy intolerant or nonresponsive to previous lactulose treatment: an open-label, pilot study. *Curr Ther Res.* 2004;65(5):413-422.
11. Leevy CB, Phillips JA. Hospitalizations during the use of rifaximin versus lactulose for the treatment of hepatic encephalopathy. *Dig Dis Sci.* 2007;52(3):737-741.
12. Bass NM, Mullen KD, Sanyal A, et al. Rifaximin treatment in hepatic encephalopathy. *N Engl J Med.* 2010;362:1071-1081.
13. Bustamante J, Rimola A, Ventura P, et al. Prognostic significance of hepatic encephalopathy in patients with cirrhosis. *J Hepatol.* 1999;30(5):890-895.
14. Adachi JA, DuPont HL. Rifaximin: a novel nonabsorbed rifamycin for gastrointestinal disorders. *Clin Infect Dis.* 2006;42(4):541-547.
15. Uribe M, Campollo I, Vargas F, et al. Acidfying enemas (lactitol and lactose) versus nonacidifying enemas (tap water) to treat acute portal-systemic encephalopathy: a double-blind, randomized clinical trial. *Hepatology.* 1987;7(4):639-643.

AUTOIMMUNE HEPATITIS
MAINTENANCE THERAPY FOR ALL PATIENTS OR STOP TREATMENT AFTER HISTOLOGIC REMISSION?

Ami Shah Behara, MD, MS; Cynthia K. Lau, MD; and David Hoffman Van Thiel, MD

Autoimmune hepatitis is a chronic immune-mediated disease that, if left untreated, has a dismal prognosis. When treated, most—but not all—patients achieve either a partial or total remission. Partial remissions generally require life-long therapy based on the concept that, off therapy, the disease will exacerbate and revert back to the poor prognosis associated with no therapy. The more critical and difficult question is: should therapy be discontinued or continued life-long on a lower maintenance immunosuppressive regiment? Discontinuation is associated with the risk of reactivation that can be severe and typically requires higher doses of the immunosuppressive agents used while continuing therapy—even at much lower doses of the immunosuppressive agent being used—is associated with readily identifiable morbidity related to the therapy rather than the primary disease. Thus the decision to either continue therapy or withdraw therapy is a critical one that requires a specific knowledge of the pathophysiology of the disease, the likelihood of reactivation, knowledge of the initial level of disease activity (grade) and its stage, the disease-related side effects experienced while receiving active therapy to achieve remission, the patient's involvement in the decision process, and the experience of the treating physician. The two polar views of this important question are addressed in the present debate.

Jensen D.
Controversies in Hepatology: The Experts Analyze Both Sides (pp 159-166)
© 2011 SLACK Incorporated

POINT

Autoimmune Hepatitis: Continue Maintenance Therapy for All Patients After Histologic Remission

by Ami Shah Behara, MD, MS

First described in 1950, autoimmune hepatitis (AIH) is a chronic liver disease with a favorable response to drug therapy but devastating consequences if left untreated. In 2010, the American Association for the Study of Liver Diseases (AASLD)[1] published clinical guidelines that defined a complete remission of AIH as disappearance of symptoms, improvement in serologic markers, and a normal liver biopsy (Table 17-1).

The pathogenesis of AIH is thought to be antibody-dependent, cell-mediated cytotoxicity associated with the presence of liver-infiltrating cytotoxic T-cells and plasma cells. This underlying pathophysiologic process cannot be altered permanently. Immunosuppressive therapy suppresses but cannot eliminate the underlying defects and subsequent cascade of immune activation that characterizes the disease. As a result, with treatment withdrawal, it is inevitable that a relapse will occur months or years later. Kirk and colleagues[2] evaluated the natural history of untreated AIH and found that over 60% of patients die within 5 years of diagnosis. These data mandate that treatment is imperative once the diagnosis of AIH is established because treatment is associated with clinical, biochemical, and histologic remission that is prolonged over several decades or more.

In 1983, Hegerty et al[3] were one of the first to examine the outcome of treatment withdrawal in patients in remission with AIH. They found that relapses occurred within 12 short weeks of treatment withdrawal (Figure 17-1). Overall, the relapse rate reported by several different groups was as high as 87%. These data document the fact that AIH is an aggressive, life-long disease process and that discontinuing maintenance therapy is fraught with considerable risk.

Multiple subsequent studies have documented further that not only does AIH relapse with treatment withdrawal, but that it occurs quickly and often and can be severe and even lethal. Montano-Loza's recent report of 102 patients with AIH identified a relapse in 102 patients (77%) within 10 ± 2 months (median 3) after termination of treatment.[4] In 2001 Kanzler et al reported that 75% of patients experienced a relapse of AIH following treatment withdrawal with a mean time to relapse of only 15 months.[5] Data from many investigations, over many years, have documented clearly that the risk of relapse is inevitable and can occur soon after the discontinuation of therapy. In addition, the risk of relapse and the severity of a relapse increases with each subsequent treatment withdrawal. Czaja[6] found that the probability of sustaining a remission for at least 6 months after drug withdrawal decreases from 51% to 14% after the second relapse and retreatment. All of the available data clearly demonstrate that withdrawal of therapy is consistently and predictably followed by a relapse. Thus, the question arises: Why would therapy be withdrawn?

The consequences of a relapse after drug withdrawal need to be emphasized to those who choose to gamble and withdraw therapy. As noted in the AASLD practice guidelines, after withdrawal of therapy for AIH, 40% of patients will progress to cirrhosis, 25% will develop esophageal varices, and 15% will die from hepatic failure.

These adverse outcomes are prevented by continued successful therapy. Even if these adverse disease-specific problems do not occur, a major concern with withdrawal of therapy

Table 17-1.

AMERICAN ASSOCIATION FOR THE STUDY OF LIVER DISEASE PRACTICE GUIDELINES

REMISSION CRITERIA IN AUTOIMMUNE HEPATITIS

- Disappearance of symptoms.
- Normal serum bilirubin and gamma globulin levels.
- Serum aminotransferase level normal or less than twice normal.
- Normal hepatic tissue or minimal inflammation and no interface hepatitis.

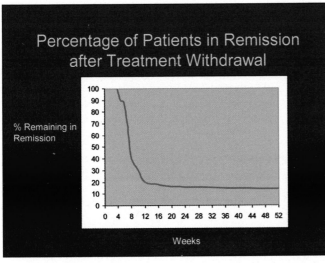

Figure 17-1. Remission after treatment withdrawal.

and a subsequent relapse is the many problems associated with retreatment. These consist of repeated courses of high-dose steroids causing potentially catastrophic side effects that include diabetes, hypertension, obesity, an increased risk of infection, osteoporosis, psychosis, gastrointestinal ulcers and bleeding, cushingoid facies, and cataract formation. These drug-related adverse effects of retreatment occur in 59% of patients who relapse. In contrast, they are rarely seen with continued low-dose maintenance therapy.

With withdrawal of therapy, one of the most frustrating concerns of health care providers is the unpredictability of who will relapse. The most disturbing fact of interruption of therapy is the report by Czaja[7] that a relapse will occur in 20% of those patients who achieved a full remission with normal hepatic architecture. Montano-Loza reported that a relapse occurs in 60%, 75%, and 74% of patients who have normal serum AST, gamma globulin, and IgG levels, respectively, at the time of withdrawal.[4] Based on current AASLD guidelines, these are the very markers that define a full disease remission. Unfortunately, patients relapse when all these criteria are met and there are no known methods to predict which patients will relapse.

The clear solution for this dilemma is maintenance immunosuppression, which is both safe and effective. Johnson et al[8] in 1995 reported the results of a clinical trial of maintenance therapy with azathioprine alone for maintenance of a clinical remission. They found that 83% of adult patients managed with azathioprine remained in remission over a median of 67 months of follow-up. Additionally, nearly half had weight loss with steroid withdrawal. Kanzler et al[5] found that patients who relapsed and those with a sustained remission were distinguishable by the duration of their prior immunosuppressive therapy. Patients with more than 4 years of continuous immunosuppressive therapy had a 67% probability of a sustained remission. More importantly, the risk of malignancy and liver-related death did not increase. These studies demonstrate that not only does maintenance therapy allow for continued remission, but that the punitive adverse effects of immunosuppression therapy are minimal in those on low-dose maintenance therapy.

Lastly, maintenance immunosuppression is inexpensive. Depending on the dose, the cost of maintenance medication is estimated to be between $120 and $430 per year. A liver biopsy, which is advocated prior to drug withdrawal per the AASLD guidelines to document histologic remission, costs upwards of $2300. This figure does not take into account the cost of any complications that may result from the procedure. Thus, the cost of a liver biopsy required to document a complete remission in an attempt to withdraw therapy is 6 to 12 times more than the cost of continued maintenance immunosuppression without accounting for additional adverse consequences.

Based upon the data presented above, it is clear that maintenance immunosuppression is superior to attempted drug withdrawal and subsequent reinstitution of high-dose therapy for a relapse and does not include the potential risk of a lethal relapse or severe exacerbation of AIH. The high frequency of relapse after treatment withdrawal mandates continued immunosuppression and avoids the problems associated with relapse that include a liver transplant for a severe relapse and potentially even death.

KEY POINTS

- The underlying pathophysiology of AIH is never eliminated with therapy; it is only controlled.
- Maintenance immunosuppression therapy is safe and effective.
- Withdrawal of maintenance immunosuppression can result in a severe exacerbation of AIH and even death.

COUNTERPOINT

Autoimmune Hepatitis: Stop Treatment After Histologic Remission?

by Cynthia K. Lau, MD

Long-term immunosuppression is not warranted in patients with AIH who experience an initial complete remission, which is defined as an asymptomatic patient with a normal serum bilirubin and aminotransferase levels that are either normal or less than 2-fold elevated, a normal IgG level, and an inactive liver histology (see Figure 17-1). According to the AASLD guidelines,[2] all adult patients should be given the opportunity to maintain their remission of AIH following discontinuation of their immunosuppressive therapy.

Currently, there are 2 different immunosuppressive regimens for adults with AIH.[9,10] These are the use of prednisone alone (20 to 60 mg per day) or combination therapy with prednisone (10 to 30 mg per day) plus azathioprine (50 mg per day). In 1975, Summerskill et al[11] reported that combination therapy with prednisone 10 mg per day plus azathioprine 50 mg per day is associated with a lower occurrence of steroid-related side effects than continued prednisone therapy alone after 1 year (10% versus 44%). Thus, they suggest that combination immunosuppressive therapy should be the preferred regimen.

There are significant well-recognized and predictable deleterious effects of long-term intermediate or high-dose corticosteroid therapy. These consist of adverse effects on linear growth and bone development; physical appearance (obesity and acne); and the presence of diabetes mellitus, hypertension, and an increased risk of opportunistic infections. Catastrophic side effects from corticosteroid use include brittle diabetes mellitus, cataracts, osteoporosis, psychosis, difficult-to-control hypertension, gastroduodenal ulcers, and severe cosmetic changes (facial rounding, dorsal hump formation, striae, profound weight gain, acne, alopecia, and facial hirsutism).[2] After 2 years of steroid therapy, regardless of the regimen, 80% of patients develop cosmetic changes. Almost half of these (44%) develop these problems within 12 months.[4] The psychological benefit of discontinuing steroid therapy is substantial, especially in young women.[5]

Another concern relative to the issue of continued treatment after a complete remission has been obtained in an individual with AIH is the hematologic side effects of azathioprine. Azathioprine use is associated with a pan-myelosuppression. In addition, it has potential teratogenic and oncogenic effects. Other identifiable complications of azathioprine therapy include cholestasis, veno-occlusive disease, nausea, vomiting, rash, pancreatitis, opportunistic infections, as well as various cytopenias and an increased risk of malignancies.[2] In 1993, Connell et al[6] evaluated the bone marrow toxicity of azathioprine in patients with inflammatory bowel disease. They found that 5% of patients manifested evidence for azathioprine-induced bone marrow toxicity and that the myelotoxicity developed randomly during treatment and could occur either suddenly or slowly over several months. Moreover, the leukopenia associated with azathioprine therapy was found to be dose dependent.

A major concern relative to the long-term consequences of immunosuppressive therapy is the increased risk of malignancy. The frequency of extrahepatic neoplasia in individuals treated for AIH is 5% after 42 months of continuous therapy. The incidence of extrahepatic malignancy is 1 per 194 patient-years of surveillance. The probability of a malignant tumor occurrence is 3% after 10 years. The risk for an extrahepatic malignancy is 1.4 fold that of an age- and sex-matched normal population. The tumors reported with azathioprine therapy have no correlation with patient age, gender, treatment regimen, or cumulative duration of treatment. Moreover, no predominant tumor type has been identified.[7]

From a review of retrospective data obtained from individuals with a variety of disease states, it has been suggested that long-term maintenance immunosuppression therapy should not be life-long, if withdrawal is possible. Permanent discontinuation of medication late in the clinical course of AIH following a relapse can be achieved in 28% of patients who relapse. There is a 47% probability of a sustained remission after initial or subsequent therapy over a 10-year period of follow-up. In 2002, Cjaza et al[8] demonstrated that conventional retreatment schedules are able to induce a sustained clinical remission more commonly than long-term maintenance schedules initiated in the absence of a remission (59% versus 12%, $P = 0.00002$). Thus, they recommend that all immunosuppressive therapy regardless of the specific agents utilized should be withdrawn following achievement of remission to assess both long-term outcome and the need for additional therapy. Potentially 25% to 30% of patients with AIH can be spared the untoward consequences of long-term immunosuppressive therapy with withdrawal of immunosuppressive therapy following achievement of a complete remission.

KEY POINTS

- Drug-free continued (long-term) remissions occur.
- Drug withdrawal avoids or reduces the immunosuppression side effects of continued therapy.
- The adverse effects of continued steroid therapy, particularly in early adolescents and young adult women, can have life-long consequences and are often psychologically damaging.

EXPERT OPINION

Continue Life-Long Therapy or Discontinue After Histologic Remission: When and How to Decide

by David Hoffman Van Thiel, MD

Autoimmune hepatitis/lupoid hepatitis (AIH) is a chronic liver disease initially described in the 1950s by several authors. Initially, it was recognized as a disease limited almost exclusively to adolescent and young adult women who presented with abnormal liver transaminases, obesity, hirsutism, hypergammaglobulinemia, antinuclear antibody positivity, and lupus erythematous prep positivity. Histologically, the disease was characterized by a lobular and periportal hepatitis with prominent piecemeal necrosis (interface hepatitis) and a leukocytic infiltrate consisting predominantly of plasma cells. On physical examination, hepatosplenomegaly was present almost universally. Moreover, advanced stage fibrosis or cirrhosis was often identified at the time of initial presentation and histologic evaluation.

With time, the disease process became recognized in both males and particularly in postmenopausal women as well as young women. The disease was found to be associated with the presence of specific HLA antigens (A3, B8, Dr3, Dr4, Dq53, and Dq54) and the presence of unique autoantibodies (soluble liver antigen, anti-neutrophil cytoplasmic antibody, antimicrosomal antibody, and antinuclear antibody). Pathophysiologically, the disease is a consequence of antibody-dependent cytotoxicity.

As a direct result of these pathologic mechanisms, immune suppression with steroids that are immunosuppressive as well as plasma cell lytic (at high dose), and more recently azathioprine, became the standard of therapy for AIH.

It soon became clear that symptomatic improvement occurred early and preceded biochemical improvement and that histologic improvement/remission occurred late, typically 2 years or more after the initiation of therapy, and was not predictable based upon the resolution of symptoms and the elimination of measures of liver injury.

The next observation relative to this disease process was that once a full remission was achieved and therapy discontinued, more than half of the patients relapsed and, worse, these relapses were often severe and required even higher doses of immunosuppression than those used prior to therapy withdrawal in order to regain control of the disease.

When one considers the numbers of patients involved (those in remission, those not achieving remission, and those that relapse), it becomes clear that only 25% to 30% of the total population remain in remission after discontinuation of therapy. As such, the question becomes: is it worth tentatively discontinuing therapy in the majority of patients (greater than 75%), who are at risk for either disease exacerbation or a severe relapse necessitating even higher doses of steroids and immunosuppression to identify the less than 25% who will remain in remission off therapy? This question is at the heart of this debate and needs to be answered by both the physician and patient when immunosuppression withdrawal is being considered. Long-term or continued therapy would appear to be the better choice, recognizing that the disease is immune-medicated and can relapse in weeks, months, and years after a remission is achieved as well as after liver transplantation.

References

1. Manns MP, Czaja AJ, Gorham JD, et al. Diagnosis and management of autoimmune hepatitis. *Hepatology.* 2010;51(6):2193-2213.
2. Kirk AP, Jain S, Pocock S, et al. Late results of the Royal Free Hospital prospective controlled trial of prednisolone therapy in hepatitis B surface antigen negative chronic active hepatitis. *Gut.* 1980;21:78-83.
3. Hegarty JE, Nouri Aria KT, Portmann B, et al. Relapse following treatment withdrawal in patients with autoimmune chronic active hepatitis. *Hepatology.* 1983;3:685-689.
4. Montano-Loza A, Carpenter HA, Czaja A. Consequences of treatment withdrawal in type 1 autoimmune hepatitis. *Liver Int.* 2007;27(4):507-515.
5. Kanzler S, Gerken G, Lohr H, et al. Duration of immunosuppressive therapy in autoimmune hepatitis. *J Hepatol.* 2001;34(2):354-355.
6. Cjaza AJ, Ammon HV, Summerskill WH. Clinical features and prognosis of severe chronic active liver disease after corticosteroid induced remission. *Gastroenterology.* 1980;78(3):518-523.
7. Cjaza AJ, Davis GL, Ludwig J, et al. Complete resolution of inflammatory activity following corticosteroid treatment of HBsAg-negative chronic active hepatitis. *Hepatology.* 1984;4:622-627.
8. Johnson PJ, McFarlane IG, Williams R. Azathioprine for long-term maintenance of remission in autoimmune hepatitis. *N Engl J Med.* 1995;333:958-963.
9. Heathcote J. Treatment strategies for autoimmune hepatitis. *Am J Gastroenterol.* 2006;101:S630-S632.
10. Al-Chalabi T, Heneghan MA. Remission in autoimmune hepatitis: what is it, and can it ever be achieved? *Am J Gastroenterol.* 2007;102:1013-1015.
11. Summerskill WH, Korman MG, Ammon HV, et al. Prednisone for chronic active liver disease: dose titration, standard dose, and combination with azathioprine compared. *Gut.* 1975;16(11):876-883.
12. Cjaza AJ. Safety issues in the management of autoimmune hepatitis. *Expert Opin Drug Saf.* 2008;7(3):319-333.
13. Connell WR, Kamm MA, Ritchie JK, et al. Bone marrow toxicity caused by azathioprine in inflammatory bowel disease : 27 years of experience. *Gut.* 1993;34(8):1081-1085.
14. Czaja AJ. Low dose corticosteroid therapy after multiple relapses of severe HBsAg-negative chronic active hepatitis. *Hepatology.* 1990;11(6):1044-1049.
15. Czaja AJ, Beaver SJ, Shiels MT. Sustained remission after corticosteroid therapy of severe hepatitis B surface antigen-negative chronic active hepatitis. *Gastroenterol.* 1987;92:215-219.

16. Wang KK, Czaja AJ, Beaver SJ, et al. Extrahepatic malignancy following long-term immunosuppressive therapy of severe hepatitis B surface antigen-negative chronic active hepatitis. *Hepatology.* 1989;10(1):39-43.

17. Kunkel HG, Ahrens EH, Eisenmenger WJ. Extreme hypergammaglobulinemia in young women with liver disease of unknown etiology. *J Clin Invest.* 1950;30:654.

18. Bearn AG, Kunkel HG, Slater RJ. The problem of chronic liver disease in young women. *Am J Med.* 1956;21(1):3-15.

19. Cowling DC, Mackay IR, Taft LI. Lupoid hepatitis. *Lancet.* 1956;271(6957):1323-1326.

20. Bartholomew LG, Hagedorn AB, Cain JC, et al. Hepatitis and cirrhosis in women with positive clot tests for lupus erythematosus. *N Engl J Med.* 1958;259(20):947-956.

21. Willocx RG, Isselbacher KJ. Chronic liver disease in young people. Clinical features and course in thirty-three patients. *Am J Med.* 1961;30:185-195.

22. Read AE, Sherlock S, Harrison CV. Active "juvenile" cirrhosis considered as part of a systemic disease and the effect of corticosteroid therapy. *Gut.* 1963;4:378-393.

23. Reynolds TB, Edmondson HA, Peters RL, et al. Lupoid hepatitis. *Ann Intern Med.* 1964;61:650-666.

24. Mistilis SP, Skyring AP, Blackburn CR. Natural history of chronic active hepatitis. I. Clinical features, course, diagnostic criteria, morbidity, mortality and survival. *Australas Ann Med.* 1968;17(3):214-223.

25. Mistilis SP, Blackburn CR. Active chronic hepatitis. *Am J Med.* 1970;48(4):484-495.

26. Machlachlan MJ, Rodnan GP, Cooper WM, et al. Chronic active ("lupoid") hepatitis; a clinical, serological, and pathological study of 20 patients. *Ann Intern Med.* 1965;62:425-462.

27. Lebovics E, Schaffner F, Klion FM, et al. Autoimmune chronic active hepatitis in postmenopausal women. *Dig Dis Sci.* 1985;30(9):824-828.

28. Mackay IR, Whittingham S, Matthews JD, et al. Genetic determinants of autoimmune chronic active hepatitis. *Springer Seminars in Immunopathology.* 1980;3(3):285-296.

29. Jensen DM, McFarlane IG, Portmann BS, et al. Detection of antibodies directed against a liver-specific membrane lipoprotein in patients with acute and chronic active hepatitis. *N Engl J Med.* 1978;299:1-7.

30. Hodgson HJ, Wands JR, Isselbacher KJ. Alteration in suppressor cell activity in chronic active hepatitis. *Proc Natl Acad Sci.* 1978;75(3):1549-1553.

31. Mieli-Vergani G, Eddleston ALWF. Autoimmunity to liver membrane antigens in acute and chronic hepatitis. *Clin Immun Aller.* 1981;1:181-197.

32. Mackay IR. Immunologic aspects of chronic active hepatitis. *Hepatology.* 1983;3(5):724-728.

33. Vento S, Nouri-Aria KT, Eddleston AL. Immune mechanisms in autoimmune chronic active hepatitis. *Scand J Gastroenterol (Suppl).* 1985;114:91-103.

34. Gurian LE, Rogoff TM, Ware AJ, et al. The immunologic diagnosis of chronic active "autoimmune" hepatitis: distinction from systemic lupus erythematosus. *Hepatology.* 1985;5(3):397-402.

35. Meyer zum Büschenfelde KH, Miescher PA. Liver specific antigens: purification and characterization. *Clin Exp Immnol.* 1972;10(1):89-102.

36. Cook GC, Mulligan R, Sherlock S. Controlled prospective trial of corticosteroid therapy in active chronic hepatitis. *Q J Med.* 1971;40:159-185.

37. Soloway RD, Summerskill WH, Baggenstoss AH, et al. Clinical, biochemical, and histological remission of severe chronic active liver disease: a controlled study of treatments and early prognosis. *Gastroenterology.* 1972;63(5):820-833.

38. Murray-Lyon IM, Stern RB, Williams R. Controlled trial of prednisone and azathioprine in active chronic hepatitis. *Lancet.* 1973;1:735-737.

39. Neuberger J, Portmann B, Calne R, et al. Recurrence of autoimmune chronic active hepatitis following orthotopic liver grafting. *Transplantation.* 1984;37:363-365.

FINANCIAL DISCLOSURES

Tarek I. Abu-Rajab Tamimi, MD has no financial or proprietary interest in the materials presented herein.

Payam Afshar, MD has no financial or proprietary interest in the materials presented herein.

Parul Dureja Agarwal, MD has not disclosed any relevant financial relationships.

Joseph Ahn, MD, MS has no financial or proprietary interest in the materials presented herein.

Andrew Aronsohn, MD has no financial or proprietary interest in the materials presented herein.

Ashley Barnabas, MD has no financial or proprietary interest in the materials presented herein.

Ami Behara, MD has no financial or proprietary interest in the materials presented herein.

Boris Blechacz, MD, PhD has no financial or proprietary interest in the materials presented herein.

Robert S. Brown Jr, MD, MPH has no financial or proprietary interest in the materials presented herein.

Thomas A. Brown, MD has no financial or proprietary interest in the materials presented herein.

James R. Burton Jr, MD has no financial or proprietary interest in the materials presented herein.

Andres F. Carrion, MD has no financial or proprietary interest in the materials presented herein.

Roger W. Chapman, MD, FRCP has no financial or proprietary interest in the materials presented herein.

Stanley Martin Cohen, MD has no financial or proprietary interest in the materials presented herein.

Neil Crittenden, MD has no financial or proprietary interest in the materials presented herein.

Brett E. Fortune, MD has no financial or proprietary interest in the materials presented herein.

Guadalupe Garcia-Tsao, MD has no financial or proprietary interest in the materials presented herein.

Leila Gobejishvili, PhD has no financial or proprietary interest in the materials presented herein.

Tyralee Goo, MD has no financial or proprietary interest in the materials presented herein.

Gregory J. Gores, MD has no financial or proprietary interest in the materials presented herein.

Dr. JS Halliday, MBBS (Hons.), FRACP has no financial or proprietary interest in the materials presented herein.

A. James Hanje, MD has no financial or proprietary interest in the materials presented herein.

Donald M. Jensen, MD is a consultant for Abbott, Boehringer-Ingelheim, BMS, Merck, Pfizer, Pharmasset, Roche, Genentech, Tibotec, and Vertex and receives research grants from Abbott, Boehringer-Ingelheim, Pharmasset, Roche, Genentech, and Tibotec.

Vandana Khungar, MD, MSc has no financial or proprietary interest in the materials presented herein.

Carmen Landaverde, MD has no financial or proprietary interest in the materials presented herein.

Cynthia K. Lau, MD has no financial or proprietary interest in the materials presented herein.

William M. Lee, MD receives consulting fees from Cumberland Pharmaceuticals.

AnnMarie Liapakis, MD has no financial or proprietary interest in the materials presented herein.

Michael Ronan Lucey, MD has not disclosed any relevant financial relationships.

Paul Martin, MD is an investigator for Genetech.

Alvaro Martinez-Camacho, MD has no financial or proprietary interest in the materials presented herein.

Craig J. McClain, MD has no financial or proprietary interest in the materials presented herein.

Anthony Michaels, MD has no financial or proprietary interest in the materials presented herein.

Arjmand R. Mufti, MD, MRCP has no financial or proprietary interest in the materials presented herein.

Kevin D. Mullen, MD is a consultant for and on the Speakers' Bureau of Salix.

Hector Nazario, MD has no financial or proprietary interest in the materials presented herein.

Neehar D. Parikh, MD has no financial or proprietary interest in the materials presented herein.

Robert Perrillo, MD is a paid consultant for Hoffman La Roche and is on the Gilead Speaker's Bureau and the Bristol Myers Squibb Speaker's Bureau.

Anjana Pillai, MD has no financial or proprietary interest in the materials presented herein.

Paul J. Pockros, MD has no financial or proprietary interest in the materials presented herein.

Fred Poordad, MD is a consultant to Merck, Vertex, Abbott, Gilead, Achillion, Genetech, and Tibotec and received payment from Merck for the development of an educational presentation.

Nataliya Razumilava, MD has no financial or proprietary interest in the materials presented herein.

Nancy Reau, MD is a paid consultant for Roche Consultation.

Mary E. Rinella, MD has no financial or proprietary interest in the materials presented herein.

Cristina Ripoll, MD has no financial or proprietary interest in the materials presented herein.

Seth N. Sclair, MD has no financial or proprietary interest in the materials presented herein.

Puneeta Tandon, MD has no financial or proprietary interest in the materials presented herein.

David Hoffman Van Thiel, MD has no financial or proprietary interest in the materials presented herein.

Lisa VanWagner, MD has no financial or proprietary interest in the materials presented herein.

Julia Wattacheril, MD, MPH has no financial or proprietary interest in the materials presented herein.

Jeffrey Weissman, MD has no financial or proprietary interest in the materials presented herein.

INDEX

AASLD. *See* American Association for the Study of Liver Diseases (AASLD)

adenomas, resection versus observation for, 93-99
  expert opinion, 97-98
  point and counterpoint, 93-96

alanine aminotransferase (ALT) levels, in hepatitis B, 34-40, 112

alcoholic liver disease
  pentoxifylline versus steroids for alcoholic hepatitis
    expert opinion, 7-8
    point and counterpoint, 3-7
  recent alcohol use in liver transplant candidates, 103-109
    expert opinion, 107-108
    point and counterpoint, 104-107
  retransplantation outcomes, 62

American Association for the Study of Liver Diseases (AASLD)
  antiviral therapy for decompensated hepatitis C cirrhotics, 44, 46
  pentoxifylline versus steroids for alcoholic hepatitis, 7, 8
  surveillance of cholangiocarcinoma in PSC patients, 150-151
  sustained virologic response as indication of cure in hepatitis C, 74
  therapy for autoimmune hepatitis in remission, 159-162
  treatment selection for hepatitis B, 35-36, 38-39
  ursodiol therapy for primary sclerosing cholangitis, 142

American College of Gastroenterology (ACG), 7, 8

antiviral therapy for hepatitis B, assessment of fibrosis for, 34, 37, 40

antiviral therapy for hepatitis C
  decompensated cirrhotics, antiviral treatment for, 43-49
    expert opinion, 49
    point and counterpoint, 43-48
  renal transplant candidates, 51-59
    expert opinion, 57
    point and counterpoint, 51-56
  retreatment in prior PEG/RBV nonresponders, 63, 65, 66, 68-69

Asian Pacific Association for the Study of the Liver (APASL), 39

asymptomatic hepatic adenoma, resection versus observation for, 93-99
  expert opinion, 97-98
  point and counterpoint, 93-96

autoimmune hepatitis
  biopsy for nonalcoholic fatty liver disease patients, 119
  living donor liver transplantation for acute liver failure, 20-24
  N-acetylcysteine for acute liver failure, 13
  remission, treatment versus nontreatment for, 159-166
    expert opinion, 164
    point and counterpoint, 159-163
  retransplantation outcomes, 62, 63, 68

azathioprine, 161-164

beta-blocker therapy, sequential portal pressure measurements for, 123-131
  expert opinion, 128-130
  point and counterpoint, 124-128

biomarkers
  assessment of fibrosis in hepatitis B, 33-40
  nonalcoholic fatty liver disease, 115-118
  pentoxifylline versus steroids for alcoholic hepatitis, 3-7

primary sclerosing cholangitis
cholangiocarcinoma detection, 151
ursodiol therapy, efficacy of, 134, 137-140
biopsy
antiviral treatment in recurrent hepatitis C, 63-65, 70
antiviral treatment of hepatitis C in renal transplant candidates, 53, 57
autoimmune hepatitis in remission, therapy for, 160, 161, 164
hepatitis B, assessment of fibrosis in, 33-42
expert opinion, 38-40
point and counterpoint, 33-38
living donor liver transplantation candidates exceeding Milan criteria, 89
nonalcoholic fatty liver disease, 111-122
expert opinion, 117-119
point and counterpoint, 111-116
primary sclerosing cholangitis, difficulties studying, 135
blood tests. *See* serological tests
Busuttil and Ghobrial score, 63, 66

CA 19-9 for cholangiocarcinoma surveillance, 145-152
expert opinion, 150-151
point and counterpoint, 146-150
cAMP (cyclic adenosine monophosphate), 4, 8
cancer. *See* cholangiocarcinoma (CCA); hepa-to-cellular carcinoma (HCC)
center experience, 26, 28, 29, 130
cGMP (guanosine cyclic monophosphate), 4
chemoprotective effects of ursodiol therapy, 136, 137, 140-143
Child-Pugh score, 45-47, 63, 66, 69, 104, 129
cholangiocarcinoma (CCA)
annual screening, need for, 145-152
expert opinion, 150-151
point and counterpoint, 146-150
ursodiol therapy, efficacy of, 135-136, 139-143
chronic kidney disease, hepatitis C treatment for renal transplant candidates, 51-59
expert opinion, 57
point and counterpoint, 51-56
cirrhosis
autoimmune hepatitis in remission, therapy for, 160

beta-blocker therapy, measurements of, 123-125, 128-129
hepatitis B virus, 34, 36, 38, 40
hepatitis C virus
decompensation, antiviral therapy for, 43-49
recurrent, retransplantation for, 62, 66-68
renal transplant candidates, 57
retreatment in PEG/RBV nonresponders, 68-69
sustained virologic response as indication of cure, 74, 75, 78
lactulose or rifaximin for hepatic encepha-lopathy, 155
nonalcoholic fatty liver disease, biopsy for, 111-113, 115, 117-119
recent alcohol use in liver transplant candi-dates, 104-106
ursodiol therapy for primary sclerosing chol-angitis, 133, 134
coercion, 19, 20, 23-25, 27, 29
coinfections, liver biopsy for, 34, 37, 38
corticosteroids. *See* steroids
cost effectiveness
assessment of fibrosis in hepatitis B, 34, 35, 39, 40
biopsy for nonalcoholic fatty liver disease, 115-117
hepatic venous pressure gradient measure-ment, 128, 129
lactulose or rifaximin for hepatic encepha-lopathy, 154-157
retransplantation for recurrent HCV with failed PEG/RBV, 62, 67, 69
screening for cholangiocarcinoma, 147, 150, 151
therapy for autoimmune hepatitis in remis-sion, 161
cyclic adenosine monophosphate (cAMP), 4, 8
cytokeratin 18, 115, 118

DAAs (direct-acting antivirals), 48, 57, 68, 69
de novo glomerulonephritis, 52, 53, 55
deceased donor liver transplantation (DDLT)
acute liver failure, 19-30
hepatocellular carcinoma beyond the Milan criteria, 84-89

decompensated liver disease
  hepatitis C virus
    antiviral therapy, 43-49
    recurrent, retransplantation for, 61, 62, 67
    sustained virologic response as indication
      of cure, 78
  living donor liver transplantation beyond the
    Milan criteria, 85, 86
  recent alcohol use in liver transplant candi-
    dates, 104-107
  surveillance of cholangiocarcinoma, 149
diagnostic scoring systems. *See* prognostic
  scoring systems
DILI (drug-induced liver injury), 13, 17
direct-acting antivirals (DAAs), 48, 57, 68, 69
donor coercion, 20, 22, 24, 25, 27-29
donor complications from living donor liver
  transplantation, 20, 22, 23, 26, 28, 29
Donor Risk Index (DRI), 63, 66, 69
dosage regimens
  antiviral therapy
    decompensated hepatitis C cirrhotics, 45-
      48
    hepatitis C in renal transplant candidates,
      53, 55-56, 57
    recurrent hepatitis C virus, 64, 65
  lactulose or rifaximin for hepatic encepha-
    lopathy, 155
  maintenance therapy for autoimmune hepa-
    titis patients, 162
  ursodeoxycholic acid, 134, 135, 137-143
DRI (Donor Risk Index), 63, 66, 69
drug-induced liver injury (DILI), 13, 17

Early Change in Bilirubin Level (ECBL), 6, 7
EASL (European Association for the Study of
  the Liver), 36, 38, 39, 142, 151
ECBL (Early Change in Bilirubin Level), 6, 7
encephalopathy
  antiviral therapy for decompensated hepatitis
    C cirrhotics, 47
  beta-blocker therapy, measurements of, 123,
    125
  lactulose or rifaximin as first-line therapy
    for, 153-158
    expert opinion, 156, 157
    point and counterpoint, 153-156
  living donor liver transplantation for acute
    liver failure, 20, 24, 25, 27

N-acetylcysteine for acute liver failure, 15
pentoxifylline versus steroids for alcoholic
  hepatitis, 6

endoscopic retrograde cholangiopancreatogra-
  phy (ERCP), 147, 149-151
European Association for the Study of the
  Liver (EASL), 36, 38, 39, 142, 151

FibroScan (transient elastography), 34, 38, 39,
  112, 113
fibrosis
  acute liver failure, 4, 5, 8, 33-34
  biopsy for assessment of, in hepatitis B, 33-
    42
    expert opinion, 38-40
    point and counterpoint, 33-38
  biopsy for nonalcoholic fatty liver disease
    patients, 112-115, 117-119
  hepatitis C in renal transplant candidates,
    treatment of, 53
  retransplantation for recurrent HCV with
    failed PEG/RBV, 61-64, 66, 68, 69
  sustained virologic response as indication of
    cure in hepatitis C, 74, 75, 78
  ursodiol therapy for primary sclerosing chol-
    angitis, 134, 137, 142
fulminant hepatic failure, living donor liver
  transplantation for, 23, 27

genotypes of hepatitis C, and treatment outcomes, 44-46, 48, 55, 65, 68-70, 76
guanosine cyclic monophosphate (cGMP), 4

HBeAg-negative versus -positive patients, 34-
  36, 38-40
hepatic venous pressure gradient (HPVG) measurements for beta-blocker therapy, 123-131
  expert opinion, 128-130
  point and counterpoint, 124-128
hepatitis B virus (HBV)
  biopsy for assessment of fibrosis, 33-42
    expert opinion, 38-40
    point and counterpoint, 33-38
  living donor liver transplantation for acute
    liver failure, 20-21
  N-acetylcysteine for acute liver failure, 13,
    17

recent alcohol use in liver transplant candidates, 107

retransplantation outcomes, 62, 63, 68

hepatitis C virus (HCV)

antiviral therapy

decompensated hepatitis C cirrhotics, 43-49

renal transplant candidates, 51-57

retreatment in prior PEG/RBV nonresponders, 63, 65, 66, 68, 69

biopsy for assessment of fibrosis, 34, 37-39

living donor liver transplantation, 20, 21, 44

recent alcohol use in liver transplant candidates, 107

retransplantation for recurrent disease with failed PEG/RBV, 61-72

expert opinion, 70

point and counterpoint, 61-69

sustained virologic response as indication of cure, 73-80

expert opinion, 77-78

point and counterpoint, 73-77

hepatitis D virus (HDV), 34, 37, 38

hepatocellular carcinoma (HCC)

antiviral therapy for decompensated hepatitis C cirrhotics, 47

asymptomatic hepatic adenomas, 94, 95, 96

biopsy for assessment of fibrosis in hepatitis B, 33, 34, 36-38, 40

biopsy for nonalcoholic fatty liver disease, 113, 119

living donor liver transplantation beyond the Milan criteria, 83-91

expert opinion, 89-90

point and counterpoint, 83-88

recent alcohol use in liver transplant candidates, 104

sustained virologic response as indication of cure in hepatitis C, 74, 75, 78

HIV (human immunodeficiency virus), 34, 37, 38, 76

imaging techniques

cholangiocarcinoma, annual screening for, 145-152

expert opinion, 150, 151

point and counterpoint, 146-150

fibrosis assessment in hepatitis B, 34, 38-39

hepatic venous pressure gradient measurements, 125

nonalcoholic fatty liver disease, 112-113, 115, 117

Imax (maximum inhibition of lymphocyte proliferation), 7

immune-suppressed patients

fibrosis assessment in hepatitis B, 34, 37, 38

post-SVR relapse, 76-78

inflammatory activity

alcoholic hepatitis, 3-6, 7

biopsy for assessment of fibrosis in hepatitis B, 34, 38-40

biopsy for nonalcoholic fatty liver disease patients, 114, 115, 117-118

remission criteria for autoimmune hepatitis, 160

retransplantation for recurrent HCV with failed PEG/RBV, 63, 66

ursodiol therapy for primary sclerosing cholangitis, 134, 142

interferon therapy, safety of, 44-48, 53-56

International Liver Transplantation Society, 62, 63

lactulose or rifaximin for hepatic encephalopathy, 153-158

expert opinion, 156, 157

point and counterpoint, 153-156

LADR (Low Accelerating Dosage Regimen), 45, 46, 48

Lille Model, 6, 7

Linhares score, 63, 66

living donor liver transplantation (LDLT)

acute liver failure in adults, 19-30

expert opinion, 28, 29

point and counterpoint, 20-28

antiviral therapy for decompensated hepatitis C cirrhotics, 44

hepatocellular carcinoma beyond the Milan criteria, 83-91

expert opinion, 89-90

point and counterpoint, 83-88

Low Accelerating Dosage Regimen (LADR), 45, 46, 48

LPS-induced hepatitis, 4

Maddrey Discriminant Function, 6

magnetic resonance cholangiopancreatography (MRCP), 145-152

expert opinion, 150, 151

point and counterpoint, 146-150

Markmann score, 63, 66, 69

maximum inhibition of lymphocyte proliferation (Imax), 7

Mayo PSC Risk Score, 135, 139, 140

MELD (model for end-stage liver disease) score
  antiviral therapy for decompensated hepatitis C cirrhotics, 43-48
  living donor liver transplantation for acute liver failure, 21, 22, 28, 29
  pentoxifylline versus steroids for alcoholic hepatitis, 5
  retransplantation for recurrent HCV with failed PEG/RBV, 62, 63, 66, 67, 68, 69

"Metroticket Calculator," 89

Milan criteria, living donor liver transplantation beyond, 83-91
  expert opinion, 89-90
  point and counterpoint, 83-88

MR spectroscopy, 115

MRCP. *See* magnetic resonance cholangiopancreatography (MRCP)

N-acetylcysteine (NAC) for non-acetaminophen acute liver failure, 11-17
  expert opinion, 15, 16
  point and counterpoint, 11-15

new-onset diabetes after transplantation (NODAT), 52, 53

nonalcoholic fatty liver disease (NAFLD), biopsy for, 111-122
  expert opinion, 117-119
  point and counterpoint, 111-116

nonalcoholic steatohepatitis (NASH)
  biopsy for, 111-122
    expert opinion, 117-119
    point and counterpoint, 111-116
  recent alcohol use in liver transplant candidates, 107

noninvasive surveillance
  assessment of fibrosis in hepatitis B, 33-40
  autoimmune hepatitis in remission, therapy for, 160-162
  lactulose or rifaximin for hepatic encephalopathy, 154, 157
  nonalcoholic fatty liver disease, 112, 113, 115-119
  pentoxifylline versus steroids for alcoholic hepatitis, 3-7
  primary sclerosing cholangitis

cholangiocarcinoma surveillance, 145-152
  ursodiol therapy, 134, 137-140, 142
  retransplantation for recurrent HCV with failed PEG/RBV, 62, 63, 66, 69
  sustained virologic response as indication of cure in hepatitis C, 74-78
  transient elastography (FibroScan), 34, 38, 39, 112, 113

nonselective beta-blockers. *See* beta-blocker therapy, sequential portal pressure measurements for

norUDCA (24-norursodeoxycholic acid), 142

obesity/weight loss, 34, 35, 113, 116-119

occult hepatitis C virus infection, 74-78

phosphodiesterases/pentoxifylline versus steroids for alcoholic hepatitis, 3-9
  expert opinion, 7-8
  point and counterpoint, 3-7

PNF (primary graft nonfunction), 23, 88

post-SVR "relapses," 74-78

prednisone. *See* steroids

pretransplantation therapy
  decompensated hepatitis C cirrhotics, 44-46
  hepatitis C in renal transplant candidates, 51-59
    expert opinion, 57
    point and counterpoint, 51-56

primary graft nonfunction (PNF), 23, 88

primary sclerosing cholangitis (PSC)
  annual screening for, 145-152
    expert opinion, 150, 151
    point and counterpoint, 146-150
  ursodiol therapy for, 133-144
    expert opinion, 142, 143
    point and counterpoint, 133-141

prognostic scoring systems
  antiviral therapy for decompensated hepatitis C cirrhotics, 43-48
  hepatocellular carcinoma, 83-87, 89
  living donor liver transplantation for acute liver failure, 21, 22, 28, 29
  nonalcoholic fatty liver disease, 112
  pentoxifylline versus steroids for alcoholic hepatitis, 5-7
  recent alcohol use in liver transplant candidates, 108
  retransplantation for recurrent HCV with failed PEG/RBV, 62, 63, 66-69

ursodiol therapy for primary sclerosing cholangitis, 135, 138-140

protease inhibitors, 48, 57, 63, 66, 68, 69

psychological effects of living donor liver transplantation, 22, 25, 27, 29, 88

PTX (pentoxifylline) versus steroids for alcoholic hepatitis, 3-9

recurrent disease
  autoimmune hepatitis in remission, treatment versus nontreatment for, 159-166
    expert opinion, 164
    point and counterpoint, 159-163
  cholangiocarcinoma, 149, 150
  hepatic encephalopathy, 154-157
  hepatitis C in decompensated cirrhotics, 44, 46
  hepatitis C in immune-suppressed patients, 76-78
  hepatocellular carcinoma, 86-89

retransplantation for recurrent HCV with failed PEG/RBV, 61-72
  expert opinion, 70
  point and counterpoint, 61-69

renal protective effect of pentoxifylline for alcoholic hepatitis, 4, 5

renal transplantation, treatment of hepatitis C prior to, 51-59
  expert opinion, 57
  point and counterpoint, 51-56

retreatment in prior PEG/RBV nonresponders, 63, 65, 66, 68, 69

ribavirin therapy, safety of, 44-48, 53, 55, 56

rifaximin or lactulose for hepatic encephalopathy, 153-158
  expert opinion, 156, 157
  point and counterpoint, 153-156

Rosen (R) score, 63, 66, 69

scoring systems. *See* prognostic scoring systems

serological tests
  assessment of fibrosis in hepatitis B, 34-40
  autoimmune hepatitis in remission, therapy for, 160-162
  lactulose or rifaximin for hepatic encephalopathy, 154, 157
  nonalcoholic fatty liver disease, 112, 113, 118, 119
  pentoxifylline versus steroids for alcoholic hepatitis, 3-7

primary sclerosing cholangitis
  cholangiocarcinoma surveillance, 145-152
  ursodiol therapy, efficacy of, 134, 137-140, 142
  retransplantation for recurrent HCV with failed PEG/RBV, 62, 63, 66, 69

sustained virologic response as indication of cure in hepatitis C, 74-78

small duct primary sclerosing cholangitis, 140

small-for-size syndrome, 21, 22

standardization of hepatic venous pressure gradient measurements, 130

steatosis, differential diagnosis of, 112-115, 117-119

steroids
  autoimmune hepatitis in remission, treatment decisions for, 159-166
    expert opinion, 164
    point and counterpoint, 159-163
  versus pentoxifylline for alcoholic hepatitis
    expert opinion, 7-8
    point and counterpoint, 3-7
  recent alcohol use in liver transplant candidates, 106, 107
  resistance/responsiveness to, 6-8, 106, 107

SVR (sustained virologic response)
  decompensated hepatitis C cirrhotics, 43-46, 48
  as indication of cure in hepatitis C, 73-80
    expert opinion, 77-78
    point and counterpoint, 73-77
  renal transplant candidates with hepatitis C, 52-56
  retransplantation for recurrent HCV with failed PEG/RBV, 63-65, 68-69

theophylline, 7, 8

transient elastography (FibroScan), 34, 38, 39, 112, 113

ultrasound, 112, 117, 125, 151

University of California, San Francisco criteria, 84-87, 89

ursodiol therapy for primary sclerosing cholangitis, 133-144
  expert opinion, 142, 143
  point and counterpoint, 133-141

variceal hemorrhage, prophylaxis of
  autoimmune hepatitis in remission, therapy
    for, 160
  biopsy for nonalcoholic fatty liver disease,
    113, 119
  sequential portal pressure measurements for
    beta-blocker therapy, 123-131
      expert opinion, 128-130
      point and counterpoint, 124-128
viral replication, 34, 40, 73, 76-78

WAIT
...There's More!

The exciting and unique Curbside Consultation Series is designed to effectively provide gastroenterologists with practical, to the point, evidence based answers to the questions most frequently asked during informal consultations between colleagues.

Each specialized book included in the Curbside Consultation Series offers quick access to current medical information with the ease and convenience of a conversation. Expert consultants who are recognized leaders in their fields provide their advice, preferences, and solutions to 49 of the most frequent clinical dilemmas in gastroenterology.

Curbside Consultation of the Colon:
49 Clinical Questions
Brooks D. Cash MD, FACP, CDR, MC, USN
208 pp., Soft Cover, 2009,
ISBN 13 978-1-55642-831-9, Order #78316, **$83.95**

Curbside Consultation in Endoscopy:
49 Clinical Questions
Joseph Leung MD and Simon Lo MD
250 pp., Soft Cover, 2009,
ISBN 13 978-1-55642-817-3, Order #78170, **$83.95**

Curbside Consultation in GERD:
49 Clinical Questions
Philip O. Katz MD
192 pp., Soft Cover, 2008,
ISBN 13 978-1-55642-818-0, Order #78189, **$83.95**

Curbside Consultation in GI Cancer for the Gastroenterologist:
49 Clinical Questions
Douglas G. Adler MD
288 pp., Soft Cover, 2011,
ISBN 13 978-1-55642-984-2, Order #79842, **$83.95**

Curbside Consultation in IBD:
49 Clinical Questions
David Rubin MD; Sonia Friedman MD; Francis A. Farraye MD
240 pp., Soft Cover, 2009,
ISBN 13 978-1-55642-856-2, Order #78562, **$83.95**

Curbside Consultation in IBS:
49 Clinical Questions
Brian E. Lacy PhD, MD
296 pp., Soft Cover, 2011,
ISBN 13 978-1-55642-985-9, Order #79859, **$83.95**

Curbside Consultation of the Liver:
49 Clinical Questions
Mitchell L. Shiffman MD
272 pp., Soft Cover, 2008,
ISBN 13 978-1-55642-815-9, Order #78154, **$83.95**

Curbside Consultation of the Pancreas:
49 Clinical Questions
Scott Tenner MD, MPH; Alphonso Brown MD, MS Clin Epi; Frank Gress MD
272 pp., Soft Cover, 2010,
ISBN 13 978-1-55642-814-2, Order #78146, **$83.95**

Please visit

www.slackbooks.com

to order any of these titles!
24 Hours a Day...7 Days a Week!

Attention Industry Partners!

Whether you are interested in buying multiple copies of a book, chapter reprints, or looking for something new and different— we are able to accommodate your needs.

Multiple Copies

At attractive discounts starting for purchases as low as 25 copies for a single title, SLACK Incorporated will be able to meet all of your needs.

Chapter Reprints

SLACK Incorporated is able to offer the chapters you want in a format that will lead to success. Bound with an attractive cover, use the chapters that are a fit specifically for your company. Available for quantities of 100 or more.

Customize

SLACK Incorporated is able to create a specialized custom version of any of our products specifically for your company.

Please contact the Marketing Communications Director of Health Care Books and Journals for further details on multiple copy purchases, chapter reprints or custom printing at 1-800-257-8290 or 1-856-848-1000.

*Please note all conditions are subject to change.

CODE: 328

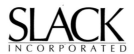

SLACK Incorporated • Health Care Books and Journals
6900 Grove Road • Thorofare, NJ 08086

1-800-257-8290 or 1-856-848-1000

Fax: 1-856-848-6091 • E-mail: orders@slackinc.com • Visit: www.slackbooks.com